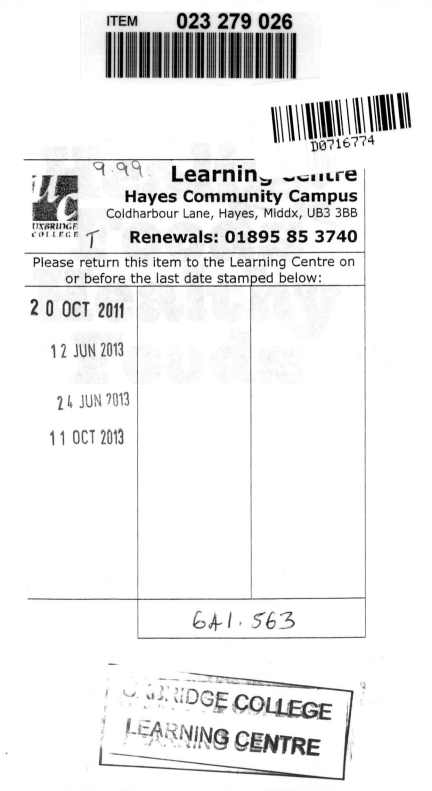

Visit our How To website at www.howto.co.uk

At **www.howto.co.uk** you can engage in conversation with our authors – all of whom have 'been there and done that' in their specialist fields. You can get access to special offers and additional content but most importantly you will be able to engage with, and become a part of, a wide and growing community of people just like yourself.

At **www.howto.co.uk** you'll be able to talk and share tips with people who have similar interests and are facing similar challenges in their lives. People who, just like you, have the desire to change their lives for the better – be it through moving to a new country, starting a new business, growing their own vegetables, or writing a novel.

At **www.howto.co.uk** you'll find the support and encouragement you need to help make your aspirations a reality.

How To Books strives to present authentic, inspiring, practical information in their books. Now, when you buy a title from **How To Books**, you get even more than just words on a page.

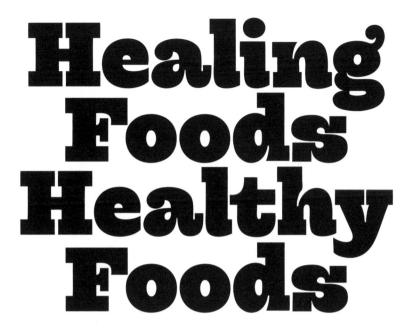

Healing Foods Healthy Foods

Using superfoods to help fight disease and maintain a healthy body

Gloria Halim

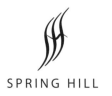

SPRING HILL

Published by Spring Hill
Spring Hill is an imprint of How To Books Ltd
Spring Hill House, Spring Hill Road,
Begbroke, Oxford OX5 1RX
Tel: (01865) 375794. Fax: (01865) 379162
info@howtobooks.co.uk
www.howtobooks.co.uk

Every effort has been made to identify and acknowledge the sources of the material quoted throughout this book. The author and publishers apologise for any errors or omissions, and would be grateful to be notified of any corrections that should appear in any reprint or new edition.

How To Books greatly reduce the carbon footprint of their books by sourcing their typesetting and printing in the UK.

First published 2011

British Library Cataloguing in Publication Data
A catalogue record for this book is available from the British Library

ISBN: 978-1-905862-53-5

Produced for How To Books by Deer Park Productions, Tavistock
Cover and text design by Anthony Prudente, Omnipress Limited, Eastbourne
Printed and bound in Great Britain by Bell & Bain Ltd, Glasgow

NOTE: The material contained in this book is set out in good faith for general guidance and no liability can be accepted for loss or expense incurred as a result of relying in particular circumstances on statements made in the book. The laws and regulations are complex and liable to change, and readers should check the current position with the relevant authorities before making personal arrangements.

Contents

Dedication and Appreciation

To God Almighty who got me through the most difficult times and made this book possible. Lord, I thank you.

I would like to thank my father for his love, strength and support. Words cannot express my gratitude. I thank God each day for keeping you healthy and strong. To my mother, you were the most kind and gentle person I've ever known and I thank God you were my mum, you taught me so much. My sister Lauretta who was there with me every step of the way, I thank you from the bottom of my heart. To my sister Valentina, who is the writer in the family, thank you for your love, support and contributions to this book. To my brother Tom and sister Felicia, thank you for the love and support, and always being there. To my brother-in-law, Najim, thank you for the support, and to my darling niece Laura, who makes me laugh and dizzy with her endless energy, I adore you. To my friends Adesua and Annie, who are more like sisters to me, thank you for all the love and support.

To all my family and friends who were there for me, and those who touched my life through this journey, too many to mention, I thank you from the bottom of my heart.

I would also like to thank Samantha Russo and Dr Keith Scott for their contributions to this book.

Foreword

It is not often that a health related book is both packed full of useful, scientifically based information as well as important practical guidance. The reason for the quality of this book is that the author, Gloria Halim is both a cancer survivor and someone who has decided to take control of her own health. By delving into the extensive body of research that shows how diet is often the deciding factor between health and disease she has produced an excellent, accessible nutritional guide.

There is still a lot of confusion about diet and its value in the prevention and management of serious diseases such as cancer. In this context *Healing Foods, Healthy Foods* is a welcome and progressive addition to the self-help health literature. This valuable book provides for both those who already have a serious disease, such as cancer, as well as for individuals who are looking for a dietary scheme that will help prevent them from falling prey to that or other illness.

What is so refreshing about Gloria's book is that it focuses on the nutritional value of a wide variety of foods; rather than providing a litany of vitamin and mineral supplements for each and every disease. The value of this approach cannot be over stated as it emphasizes the importance of selecting a core group of nutrient-rich foods that provides a full range of dietary compounds known to be essential for good health.

I was even more impressed to see that the super foods chapter focuses on widely available and affordable fruits, vegetables, pulses, herbs and spices. Thankfully Gloria has avoided the temptation to include in this chapter a preponderance of rare and expensive foods that are obtainable only from specialty outlets.

Gloria saves the best part of *Healing Foods, Healthy Foods* for the final section of the book where she provides us with a wonderful selection of mouth watering recipes. These recipes bring her previous chapters to life and show that, with the right advice, healthy eating should also be a gourmet experience. Moreover her liberal use of herbs and spices in all of the recipe categories will warm your heart, delight your taste buds and give your health a considerable boost.

Healing Foods, Healthy Foods is a book that is exactly what is needed at this time. We should all be grateful to Gloria for devoting herself and her resources to the research and effort required to produce such a wonderful publication.

Dr Keith Scott
Medical doctor and author of *Medicinal Seasonings, The Healing Power of Spices* Cape Town, South Africa

About
Samantha Russo

Samantha Russo, who wrote Chapter 5, who is a qualified Nutrition Advisor and swimming coach. In her early career she worked in television in South Africa and then relocated to Israel for a few years where she owned her own juice bar. She wanted to provide people with their own choices when cleansing their bodies. There isn't a lot Sami doesn't know about the benefits and properties of most fruits, vegetables, grains and seeds, herbs and spices. She is an avid believer in juicing – to get as much nutrients in as possible in the quickest, tastiest (sometimes not-so-tasty) way possible!

After moving to England she decided to put a certificate to her knowledge and studied at The Institute of Optimum Nutrition – and then obtained a Nutrition and Weight Management diploma from Future Fit. She consults on a one to one basis or with groups of people who want to lose weight and get fit and healthy. Being a swimmer herself, she is qualified to consult with athletes as well as adults and children with allergies and eating disorders.

Introduction

I would like to begin with two quotes by Wayne Dyer: 'You don't know the value of good health until you lose it' and 'Change the way you look at things and the things you look at change'. Illness has the tendency to change the way you view life and yourself.

About two years ago, I was diagnosed with breast cancer. I was at the peak of my career as an IT consultant, enjoying my work, living the city life in London and it all came to a screeching halt when I was diagnosed. I couldn't help trying to figure out what the culprit was – did bad diet play a part in it or was it down to genes? I obviously cannot change the latter but right then I wished I had been more careful with what I ate. Looking back, I realised that my diet was quite bad, in fact so bad that I had started to call myself the 'junk food queen'. My vice was sugar. I have a sweet tooth so at any given opportunity I ate chocolate, cakes of any kind, ice cream – if it was sweet I ate it. I didn't eat too much fast food and I have always eaten fruit as part of my diet so I remember thinking that as long as I ate fruit, drank loads of water and did the odd bit of exercise here and there, even though I drowned myself in loads of sweet foods I would be fine. How wrong I was. I have since found out that cancer cells feed on sugar to multiply; boy, did I have a lot of sugar in my system. I'm not saying that was the main reason for why I got cancer, but it might have been one of the factors that contributed to it.

During the course of treatment, I carried out extensive research on good foods (herbs, spices, grains, fruits, vegetables, seafood, etc.) that boost health and energy (as chemo really got the best of me…). At the time, food was revolting to me and tasted really bad as you lose your taste buds during treatment. They tell you that you need to eat to keep your strength up which was easier said than done. I found the only foods I could stomach were salads and sometimes soups, which wasn't often. It's all about going back to basics and nature: cutting out fast foods, junk and processed foods. I came up with some really good recipes (yes, tasty too), which helped boost my immune system and increase my energy levels. I also tried a lot of good recipes from the Mediterranean and Asian regions, which have been highlighted as the healthiest diets in the world, as well as from the African region. I made some of these recipes my own by changing some of the ingredients and sometimes cooking methods to suit my taste. I chose these recipes because of the ingredients – the use of a lot of herbs, spices and super foods.

This book includes these recipes as well some from family and friends who have kindly loaned them to me as I loved them so much. Eating in this way has worked and is still working for me. I have also noticed that my attitude has changed for the better. Hence, good food = fab health = positive attitude. I decided to put this all in one book because, during my research, I ended up with a lot of different books containing information about super foods, spices and oils, as well as recipe books. As I couldn't find one single book that consolidated all the information and recipes, I wrote this book, which I cannot wait to share with you.

In Chapter 5, Acid to Placid, you will find information on the benefits of keeping your body in an alkaline state. This material has been contributed by Samantha Russo, who has been a nutritionist for over ten years, and it has been tried and tested by her and her clients.

Even if you are not a cancer sufferer or survivor, this book will help you on your way to healing and improving your overall health. This is by no means an alternative to modern medicine and I don't claim to know the ins and outs of the medical profession or terminologies. I would add that you also need to exercise. Your body needs physical tuning; you take your car for a service, so why not service your body? I started yoga which I think is fantastic as there are different types and strengths; you just have to find the one which best suits you. I also walk a lot and swim. It's all about understanding and listening to what your body is telling you. Treat your body with love and it will love you back and try to keep stress at bay. The point is trying to look at ways to change your lifestyle to be healthy and less stressed out. I am now doing what I've always loved as a hobby (Interior Design) and also working on designing a lingerie line for women who have been through breast cancer which I find very fulfilling as I feel like I'm making a difference in my own little way. Most of all I thank God every day for the abundance and good health He brings into my life. Without Him, I would not be sharing this book with you.

I hope you enjoy it!

Chapter 1

Super Foods

Super foods are rich in vitamins, minerals and antioxidants. They are usually best eaten in their raw form (e.g. apples, berries, broccoli when juiced, etc.) or steamed to prevent loss of nutrients. Below is a list of super foods, along with their nutritional content and dietary uses. This can be used as a guide to help treat any ailment you may have or simply to keep your body healthy by providing it with a balanced diet.

Almonds

Almonds are a great source of vitamin E, with 25g providing 70 percent of the recommended daily allowance. They also contain good amounts of magnesium, potassium, zinc, selenium, copper, potassium, phosphorus, biotin, riboflavin, niacin, iron and fibre, and they are a good source of healthy monounsaturated fat. They contain more calcium than any other nut, which makes them great for vegans who do not eat any dairy products. They also contain amygdalin, also known as laetrile or vitamin B17, the controversial anti-cancer nutrient that some claim may contribute to fighting cancer.

Almonds contain several phytochemicals including beta-sitosterol, stigmasterol and campesterol, which is thought to contribute to a healthy heart. A handful of almonds a day helps to reduce the risk of heart disease by lowering low-density lipoprotein (LDL) or 'bad' blood cholesterol by as much as 10 percent.

Their high monounsaturated fat content, a key fat found in many Mediterranean diets, gives them much greater benefits than simply being cholesterol lowering. Nearly every research study shows that those who eat a traditional Mediterranean diet not only have a lower risk of heart disease and cancer, they also live longer.

So, what is the Mediterranean diet? This diet incorporates the basics of healthy eating with olive oil and perhaps a glass of red wine – among other components characterizing the traditional cooking style of countries that border the Mediterranean Sea. The Mediterranean diet is known to be low in saturated fat, high in monounsaturated fat and high in dietary fibre.

A recent analysis of more than 1.5 million healthy adults demonstrated that following a Mediterranean diet was associated with a reduced risk of overall and cardiovascular mortality, a reduced incidence of cancer and cancer mortality, and a reduced incidence of Parkinson's and Alzheimer's diseases.

The Mediterranean diet emphasizes getting plenty of exercise, eating primarily plant-based foods such as fruit and vegetables, whole grains, legumes and nuts; replacing butter with healthy fats such as olive oil; using herbs and spices instead of salt to flavour foods; limiting red meat to no more than a few times a month; eating fish and poultry at least twice a week; and drinking red wine in moderation. The diet also recognizes the importance of enjoying meals with family and friends.

Apples

Apples are one of nature's best 'fast' foods. The benefits supplied by apples are huge and very encouraging, and include protecting bone health, contributing to the possible prevention of asthma, heart disease and cancers such as lung, breast, colon and liver cancers. In order to get these benefits, apples need to be part of a daily healthy diet.

French researchers found that a flavonoid called phloridzin, which is found only in apples, may protect post-menopausal women from osteoporosis and may also increase bone density. Another nutrient found in apples, known as boron, also strengthens bones. New research suggests that the phytonutrient quercetin, may help to prevent Alzheimer's and Parkinson's.

The pectin in apples lowers LDL or 'bad' cholesterol. People who eat two apples per day may lower their cholesterol by as much as 16 percent. According to a study of 10,000 people, those who ate the most apples had a 50 percent lower risk of developing lung cancer. Researchers believe this is due to the high levels of the flavonoids, quercetin and naringin.

It is important to keep in mind that a lot of the goodness of this is fruit is contained in the skin. If they are not organic, they need to be washed carefully and thoroughly before being eaten whole.

Asparagus

Asparagus originates from the Mediterranean, and the southern and northern parts of Africa, with Egypt possibly being the first country to cultivate and value this vegetable for its medicinal properties.

Asparagus is a member of the lily family, which includes leeks, garlic and onions. It is an alkaline food, which is rich in protein but low in calories and carbohydrates. It is also an excellent source of potassium, folic acid, vitamins A, C and K and traces of vitamin B complex. It has an abundance of an amino acid called asparagine, which helps to cleanse the body of waste material. Some people tend to pass out smelly urine after eating asparagus. It is one of the few vegetables that are highly dense in healthful nutrients that help alleviate many ailments.

A unique phytochemical in asparagus that produces anti-inflammatory effects helps relieve arthritis and rheumatism. Asparagus is also a prime source of antioxidant and glutathione that can help prevent cancer and also the progression of cataracts and other eye problems. The healthful nutrients in asparagus juice make it an important addition to the diet of people who are trying to control their blood sugar levels. However, it is not to be taken by people with advanced kidney diseases.

Aubergines

Aubergines are part of the nightshade (Solanacene) family, which also includes tomatoes, potatoes and chilli peppers. Like all other edible members of this family, the aubergine is thought to have originated in India where it grew wild, and it was first cultivated in China. It was introduced into Europe during the Middle Ages by the Moors when it soon became popular. Thomas Jefferson introduced aubergines to the United States in 1806. It's known as eggplant in America, aubergine in Europe, and brinjal in South Africa.

Aubergine is an excellent source of dietary fibre and vitamins B1, B6 and potassium, as well as copper, magnesium, manganese, phosphorus, niacin and folic acid. In a study to determine the glycemic index (GI) of various vegetables, it was concluded that aubergine has a low GI of 15.

Aubergine has been used as a cholesterol-lowering agent, and there are some studies to support that claim. Other studies, however, do not support this so further research is needed to establish its effectiveness in lowering cholesterol.

The National Diabetes Education Program of NIH, Mayo Clinic and American Diabetes Association recommend an aubergine-based diet as a source of management for type 2 diabetes. The rationale for this suggestion is the high fibre and low soluble carbohydrate content.

The formation of new blood vessels in the body is known as angiogenesis, and is a normal process in growth and wound healing. Angiogenesis also plays an important role in the growth and spread of cancer by feeding the cancer cells with oxygen and nutrients. In a study at the Department of Nutritional Science in Japan, it was established that nasunin, the antioxidant from aubergine peel, is an angiogenesis inhibitor, and might be useful in preventing angiogenesis-related diseases.

Avocados

The story behind the avocado is that it originated in Mexico or Central and South America, and was cultivated there by the pre-Inca races of Peru, and the Mayas of Yucatan and Guatemala.

Avocados are an excellent source of monounsaturated fatty acids, potassium, vitamins E and B, and fibres. A week-long study involving 45 volunteers who ate avocados every day reported an average 17 percent drop in total cholesterol, LDL ('bad') cholesterol and triglycerides, and an 11 percent increase in high-density lipoprotein (HDL) levels. They are rich in natural beta-sitosterol, and the American Journal of Medicine has reported that researchers found that beta-sitosterol was able to lower LDL cholesterol in 16 human studies.

According to a report in the Journal of Nutritional Biochemistry, the carotenoids and tocopherols (chemical compounds which may have vitamin E activity) in avocado were shown to inhibit the growth of prostate cancer cell lines in an artificial environment (in vitro). Studies have shown that phytochemicals extracted from the avocado fruit inhibit and kill cancer cells, suggesting that the phytochemicals from avocado included in diet may offer protection against cancer.

Avocados contain glutathione, which functions as an antioxidant to scavenge free radicals, which is what we need to rid our bodies of. Dr David Heber, director of the UCLA Centre for Human Nutrition, has stated that evidence suggests that glutathione may help prevent certain types of cancers and heart disease. Three factors in avocado, folate, glutathione and potassium, help prevent high blood pressure and stroke. They also help to lower homocysteine levels, cholesterol and atherosclerosis.

According to the American Institute for Cancer Research in Washington, replacing butter, cheese or cream on a sandwich with mashed avocado not only helps to reduce calories but also increases the healthy monounsaturated fatty acids (MUFA) intake.

Avocado oil, which I call nature's cosmetic remedy, strengthens the skin by stimulating collagen, thereby reducing wrinkles and improving skin texture. Being rich in vitamin E, a free radical scavenger, it assists in slowing the aging process. Avocado oil offers better skin penetration than almond, olive and soya oils, and transports nutrients through the outer layer of the skin to the deeper layers. Who needs Botox when you have avocado oil!

Avocados are also rich in leutein and zeaxanthin, which help in the prevention of age-related macular degeneration and cataracts. In studies to determine the estimated GI of various foods, it was concluded that avocados have a low GI of 15.

Bananas

Compared to apples, bananas have twice the amount of carbohydrates, three times the amount of phosphorus, four times the amount of protein, five times the amount of vitamin A and iron, and twice the amount of other vitamins and minerals. They also naturally contain three types of sugar: sucrose, fructose and glucose. These sugars give the body an almost instant and long-lasting energy boost. Research has shown that consuming two bananas provides energy for a 90-minute workout.

Bananas have the added bonus of being rich in potassium, an essential ingredient in keeping the heart and nervous system in good shape. Potassium is essential for proper muscle contraction and thus plays an important role in muscle-influenced activities including the normal rhythmic pumping of the heart, digestion, muscular movements, etc. Some studies have also linked low potassium intake to high blood pressure and increased risk of stroke.

Bananas are one of the highest sources of naturally available vitamin B6. Vitamin B6 plays an important role in converting tryptophan (an amino acid which occurs in protein) to serotonin, and it also helps the body to produce haemoglobin. Vitamin B6 is essential for antibody production and in maintaining a healthy immune system. It also helps to convert carbohydrates to glucose, hence maintaining proper blood sugar levels.

Beans

Beans are loaded with protein and dozens of key nutrients, including a few most women fall short of, such as calcium, potassium and magnesium. 185g of beans contains 13g of fibre, which is half of what we need daily, with no saturated fat. Studies also tie beans to a reduced risk of heart disease, type 2 diabetes, high blood pressure, breast and colon cancers. An explanation of different types of beans with their benefits follows.

Mung Beans

Mung beans, also known as bean sprouts, are part of the legume family and are a good source of protein. When sprouted, mung beans contain vitamin C that is not found in the bean itself. They are rich in folic acid, iron, zinc, potassium, magnesium, copper, manganese, phosphorus and thiamine. They are also high in fibre, low in saturated fat, low in sodium and contain no cholesterol. Because of the wide range of nutrients contained in mung beans, they offer a whole host of benefits for the immune system, metabolism, heart and other organs. Include mung beans in salads or stir-fries.

Pinto Beans

Pinto beans' contribution to a healthy heart lies not just in their fibre, but in the significant amounts of antioxidants, folic acid, vitamin B6 and magnesium they supply. Folic acid and B6 help lower levels of homocysteine, an amino acid that is an intermediate product in an important metabolic process called the methylation cycle. Elevated levels of homocysteine are an independent risk factor for heart attack, stroke or peripheral vascular disease, and are found in between 20 to 40 percent of patients with heart disease.

Including pinto beans in diet may help protect against cancer. In one analysis of dietary data collected by validated food frequency questionnaires in 1991 and 1995 from 90,630 women in the Nurses' Health Study II, researchers found a significant reduced frequency of breast cancer in those women who consumed a higher intake of common beans or lentils. Eating beans two or more times per week was associated with a 24 percent reduced risk of breast cancer. For people like me who don't like beans, this would take a lot of getting used to.

Black-eyed Beans

Black-eyed beans have a smooth texture, pea-like flavour and are good when mixed with other vegetables. Like most beans, black-eyed beans are rich in soluble fibre, which helps eliminate cholesterol from the body. They are a good source of folate, potassium, copper, phosphorus and manganese. As a high potassium, low sodium food, they help reduce high blood pressure. Not only are they low in fat but, when combined with grains, beans supply high quality protein which provides a healthy alternative to meat or other animal protein. Beans also contain protease inhibitors, which slow the development of cancerous cells.

Kidney Beans

Kidney beans, like all other beans discussed above, are a very good source of cholesterol-lowering fibre. In addition, kidney beans' high fibre content prevents blood sugar levels from rising too rapidly after a meal, making them an especially good choice for people with diabetes, insulin resistance or hypoglycaemia. When combined with whole grains such as rice, they provide virtually fat-free, high quality protein.

Kidney beans are an excellent source of the trace mineral, molybdenum, an integral part of the enzyme sulfite oxidase, which is responsible for detoxifying sulfites. Sulfites are a type of preservative commonly added to prepared foods like salads.

Berries

Berries contain phytochemicals and flavonoids that may help prevent some forms of cancer. Eating a diet rich in blackberries, blueberries, raspberries, cranberries and strawberries may help to reduce the risk of several types of cancers. Blueberries and raspberries also contain lutein, which is important for healthy nutrients.

Berries are packed full of vitamins, minerals and fibre. Many of their phytonutrients, such as anthocyanins, quercetin and ellagic acid, have an antioxidant effect. They counter the natural oxidation in the body that contributes to the aging of tissues and many degenerative illnesses such as cancer, dementia and damage to the arteries.

Berries tend to spoil quickly, especially if they're broken or stored in damp conditions. Before buying, check them carefully for mould or broken berries. Also, don't rinse your berries until you're ready to eat them. If you can't eat them within a day or two, either freeze them or cook them into a sauce, which can be refrigerated for up to a week. Freezing and cooking do not damage most of the phytochemicals in the fruit, although cooking lowers the vitamin C content.

Bok Choy

Many of us probably omit this vegetable, also known as Pak Choy, in favour of more familiar forms of cabbage and greens, mostly because we don't know what to do with it. However, overlooking bok choy would be a mistake because this super Asian vegetable has a number of useful health benefits and is rich with vitamins and minerals essential for healthy living.

Also known as Chinese white cabbage, among other names, it is frequently found with wonton soup and many stir-fry dishes offered in Japanese and Chinese restaurants and it is crunchy when stir-fried. Mildly flavoured with a tender sweetness, it is a welcome accompaniment to many meals without being overpowering. It can be found fresh all year round.

This leafy vegetable is low in fat and calories and has a low carbohydrate content. It also contains potassium and vitamin B6. The rich amount of beta-carotene in this super vegetable can help to reduce the risk of certain cancers. Beta-carotene, also found in cabbage and carrots, has also been known to reduce the risk of cataracts. It is also an excellent source of folic acid and contains other healthy nutrients such as iron.

Bok choy is a rich source of many essential vitamins such as A, C and K. Vitamin A is essential for proper functioning of the immune system, improvement of vision and growth of bones and teeth. Vitamin K plays a significant role in the coagulation of blood and also facilitates the absorption of calcium and maintains bone density. Vitamin C is well known for its natural antioxidant properties, which protects the body from harmful effects of free radicals.

It is a rich source of vitamin D, which facilitates the absorption of calcium and phosphorus, and thereby ensures healthy bones and teeth. Bok choy provides sufficient amounts of folate and vitamin B6. Folate is mainly required for proper development of tissues and cells and is associated with lowering the risk of heart diseases. Vitamin B6, on the other hand, is crucial for carbohydrate, fat and protein metabolism and formation of red blood cells and antibodies.

Broccoli

Not only is broccoli an excellent source of fibre, but half of its fibre is insoluble and the other half soluble, helping to meet the needs for both types of fibre. Broccoli provides a health bonus in the form of protective substances that may shield you from diseases.

It belongs to the cabbage family known as cruciferous vegetables and health organizations have singled out cruciferous vegetables as must have foods, recommending we eat them several times a week because they are linked to lower rates of cancer. Like all cruciferous vegetables, broccoli naturally contains two important phytochemicals, indoles and isothiocyanates. Researchers at the John Hopkins University School of Medicine in Baltimore isolated from broccoli an isothiocyanate, called sulforaphane, which increases the activity of a group of enzymes in our bodies that kill cancer-causing agents.

Broccoli provides a high amount of vitamin C, which aids iron absorption in the body, prevents the development of cataracts and also eases the symptoms of the common cold. The folic acid in broccoli helps women sustain normal tissue growth and is often used as a supplement when taking birth control pills and during pregnancy. The potassium in broccoli aids those battling high blood pressure, while a large amount of calcium helps combat osteoporosis.

Brussels Sprouts

Brussels sprouts are loaded with vitamin A, folacin, potassium and calcium. They are very high in fibre and belong to the disease-fighting cabbage family. Like broccoli and cabbage, fellow cruciferous vegetables, brussels sprouts contain a phytochemical known as indole, which may help protect against cancer.

Brussels sprouts are also rich in vitamin C, another anti-cancer agent. The health benefits of this vegetable are remarkable: it boosts immune function, strengthens the heart and capillaries and helps lessen asthma symptoms. Brussels sprouts are high in vitamins A, K and B6, and are a good source of folate, fibre, potassium, phytonutrients and antioxidants. They are high in complex carbohydrates, low in fat and cholesterol and are one of the few vegetables that have over 2 grams of protein per serving.

One of the most important features of this vegetable is its ability to reduce the risk of many types of cancer including lung, colorectal, prostate and breast cancers. In addition, brussels sprouts may help prevent strokes, hypothyrodism and cataracts. A diet high in brussels sprouts can also lower the chance of developing multiple sclerosis, high blood pressure and diabetes.

Another unique characteristic of brussels sprouts and other cruciferous vegetables such as cabbage, cauliflower, broccoli and kale are their high sulforaphane content. Sulforaphane is a phytonutrient that is formed when cruciferous vegetables are chopped or chewed. It triggers the liver to produce enzymes that detoxify cancer-causing agents. The phytonutrients in brussels sprouts and other cruciferous vegetables actually signal our genes to increase production of enzymes involved in detoxification and help clear potentially carcinogenic substances more quickly than any other vegetable.

Bulghur

The health benefits of bulghur wheat include helping to prevent constipation and cancer and reducing the risk of diabetes and heart disease. Bulghur contains a compound called ferulic acid which can prevent nitrates and nitrites, common in many foods, from converting into nitrosamines, which have been linked to cancer. Bulghur wheat also contains lignans, which are considered cancer warriors due to their high antioxidant properties. These super healthy lignans also prevent cholesterol from being damaged by free radicals which makes it easier to stick to the arterial walls. Less cholesterol on the artery walls means less chance of developing heart disease.

A diet rich in bulghur wheat also adds more fibre that not only provides more heart disease, diabetes and cancer prevention, but the insoluble fibre it contains helps eliminate waste from the body faster, making it helpful in preventing and treating constipation, diverticular disease, haemorrhoids and intestinal polyps.

Bulghur wheat also has one of the highest mineral contents of any food. It is rich in iron, phosphorus, zinc, manganese, selenium and magnesium. It is the perfect addition to any meal that is high in nitrates.

Butternut Squash

Butternut squash is low in fat and delivers an ample dose of dietary fibre, making it an exceptionally heart-friendly choice. It provides significant amounts of potassium important for healthy bones and vitamin B6 essential for the proper functioning of both the nervous and immune systems. The folate content adds yet another boost to its heart-healthy reputation and helps guard against brain and spinal cord-related birth defects such as spina bifida.

The colour of butternut squash signals an abundance of powerhouse nutrients known as carotenoids, shown to protect against heart disease. In particular, the gourd boasts very high levels of beta-carotene, identified as a deterrent against breast cancer and age-related macular degeneration, as well as being a supporter of healthy lung development in foetuses and newborns. It is also rich in vitamin C and may have anti-inflammatory effects because it is rich in antioxidants.

Cabbage

Cabbage is a good source of vitamins C and B6, potassium, folic acid, biotin, calcium, magnesium and manganese. Studies have indicated that increased cabbage intake may inhibit the metastatic capacity of breast cancer (i.e. that it may inhibit the spread of cancer cells in other parts of the body), and cruciferous vegetable intake may reduce breast cancer risk. Other research data provides strong evidence for a substantial protective effect of cruciferous vegetable consumption on lung cancer and it has been associated with a decrease in gastrointestinal, prostate and bladder cancers. The anti-cancer properties of cabbage are due to its phytochemical compounds called glucosinolates, which work primarily by increasing antioxidant defence mechanisms, as well as by improving the body's ability to detoxify and eliminate harmful chemical hormones.

Cabbage is a good source of the amino acid glutamine, which increases the body's ability to secrete human growth hormone (HGH). Glutamine also has anti-inflammatory properties and assists with immune system regulation and intestinal health. Research at the Stanford University School of Medicine demonstrated that fresh cabbage juice is extremely effective in the treatment of peptic ulcers.

Carrots

Carrot is a root vegetable that offers a good source of antioxidants. It is known scientifically as Daucus Carota. Carrots are rich in vitamins A, C and K, and potassium. They help in reducing cholesterol, aid in the prevention of heart attack and in warding off certain cancers. Most of the benefits of carrots are attributed to their beta-carotene and fibre content.

British researchers discovered that increasing beta-carotene consumption from 1.7 to 2.7 milligrams a day reduced lung cancer risk by more than 40 percent. The average carrot contains about three milligrams of beta-carotene. In a study, researchers at the Danish Institute of Agricultural Sciences found that a substance called falcarinol found in carrots has been found to reduce the risk of a wide range of cancers. Another study shows that women who ate raw carrots were five to eight times less likely to develop breast cancer than women who did not eat carrots.

Carrots have antiseptic properties and therefore can be used as a laxative, vermicide and as a remedy for liver conditions. Carrot oil is good for dry skin. It makes the skin softer, smoother and firmer. Carrot juice improves stomach and gastrointestinal health.

Cauliflower

Cauliflower is a cruciferous vegetable containing many of the same cancer fighting properties as broccoli, kale and cabbage, which have become poster children for cancer prevention. The isothiocyanates formed when cauliflower is chewed activate liver enzymes that detoxify cancer-causing chemicals. The isothiocyanates along with another chemical, sulforaphane, stop the proliferation of cancer cells in the laboratory. Cauliflower is also a good source of indoles. These are chemicals which subtly alter oestrogen metabolism so that weaker oestrogens are produced that are less likely to cause breast and prostate cancer.

Cauliflower is a surprisingly good source of vitamin C. A single serving of cauliflower provides over half of the recommended daily requirement of vitamin C.

Celery

Celery leaves have a high content of vitamin A, while the stems are an excellent source of vitamins B1, B2, B6 and C with rich supplies of potassium, folic acid, calcium, magnesium, iron, phosphorus, sodium and essential amino acids. Nutrients in the fibre are released during juicing, aiding bowel movements. The natural organic sodium (salt) in celery is safe for consumption and essential for the body. While many foods lose nutrients during cooking, most of the compounds in celery hold up well. The important minerals in this magical juice effectively balance the body's blood pH, neutralizing acidity. Celery juice acts as the perfect post-workout tonic as it replaces lost electrolytes and rehydrates the body with its rich minerals.

Celery has been known to contain eight families of anti-cancer compounds. Among them are the acetylenics that have been shown to stop the growth of tumour cells, phenolic acids which block the action of prostaglandins that encourage the growth of tumour cells, and coumarins which help free radicals from damaging cells and prevent the formation and development of stomach and colon cancers. The juice has been shown to effectively and significantly lower total cholesterol and LDL ('bad') cholesterol. The natural laxative effect of celery helps to relieve constipation. It also helps relax nerves that have been overworked by man-made laxatives.

The potassium and sodium in celery juice help to regulate body fluid and stimulate urine production, making it an important way to rid the body of excess fluid. The polyacetylene in celery is an amazing relief for all inflammation such as rheumatoid arthritis, osteoarthritis, gout, asthma and bronchitis. Celery promotes healthy and normal kidney function by aiding elimination of toxins from the body and thereby preventing the formation of kidney stones. A compound in celery juice called phtalides helps relax the muscles around the arteries, dilating the vessels and allowing the blood to flow normally, which in turn lowers blood pressure.

Chickpeas

Chickpeas (garbanzo beans or kabuli chana) belong to the class of food called legumes or pulses. They have a delicious nutty taste and buttery texture, and make tasty dishes like hummus, falafels and curried chole. They contain a good amount of molybdenum, manganese, folate, fibre and tryptophan, and provide important nutrients such as protein, copper, phosphorus and iron. The nutrition profile of chickpeas makes them an important source of protein and fibre for vegetarian diets.

Chickpeas contain phytochemicals called saponins which act as antioxidants. They help to lower cholesterol and could lower the risk of breast cancer, protect against osteoporosis and minimize hot flushes in post-menopausal women.

Chickpeas can also boost your energy levels because of their high iron content. The soluble fibre helps stabilize blood sugar levels. Including chickpeas regularly in your diet can lower LDL cholesterol. They contain significant amounts of folate and magnesium. Folate lowers the level of amino acid and homocysteine, and strengthens the blood vessels.

Citrus

The first thing that comes to mind when we think of vitamin C are various types of citrus fruit as they offer numerous health benefits. However, don't restrict citrus fruit to just the provision of vitamin C as they are also rich in other important nutrients like folate, potassium, thiamine, niacin and fibre, amongst others. Additionally, they are high in antioxidants and are fat free, sodium free and even cholesterol free.

Oranges are one of the major fruits that fall under the category of being vitamin C rich. Other citrus fruits include limes, lemons, grapefruits, tangerines, clementines, satsumas and mandarins.

Eating citrus fruit regularly can keep your heart healthy. Studies have shown that they prevent a rise in levels of oxidized LDL and also help to lower blood pressure. A growing body of research is establishing a strong role for vitamin C in protecting the body against cancer. Though the research is still not complete, there is evidence that citrus fruit helps prevent the formation of cancers, slow the growth of existing cancers, and also help in killing cancer cells already present in the body. This will be true especially for citrus fruit such as lemons and limes as they are good for cleansing the body. The acid scours the intestinal tract, eliminating toxins and neutralizing harmful bacteria.

Cloves

Cloves are the fruit of a tree indigenous to Indonesia. In addition to their culinary uses, cloves have mild analgesic properties and oil of clove has long been used in dentistry as a treatment for toothache. Cloves are loaded with many highly effective antioxidants including procyanidin and quercetin. There is also evidence that eugenol and eugenol acetate inhibit platelet aggregation and thus protect against heart attack and thrombotic stroke.

Due to its antiseptic properties, clove oil is useful for wounds, cuts, scabies, athlete's foot, fungal infections, bruises, etc. It can also be used to treat insect bites and stings. Clove oil is very strong in nature and should be diluted before using. Furthermore, it should not be used on sensitive skin. Clove oil has cooling and anti-inflammatory effects, which help in clearing the nasal passages. This expectorant is useful in various respiratory disorders including coughs, colds, bronchitis, asthma, sinusitis and tuberculosis. Chewing a clove bud eases sore throats. Both clove and clove oil are useful for boosting the immune system. Its antiviral properties and ability to purify blood increases your resistance to diseases.

Coconut

Coconut is a tropical fruit rich in protein that is found in the African, Asian and Caribbean regions and in India. The flesh of the coconut is very good for destroying intestinal parasites, which we may get from eating infected food. Coconut water is good for kidney and urinary bladder problems. Coconut oil is good for the immune system as it contains antimicrobial lipids, lauric acid, capric acid and caprylic acid, which have antifungal, antibacterial and antiviral properties. The human body converts lauric acid into monolaurin, which it is claimed helps in dealing with viruses and bacteria causing diseases such as herpes, influenza, etc.

When applied on infections, coconut oil forms a chemical layer which protects the infected body part from external dust, air, fungi, bacteria and virus. It is most effective on bruises as it speeds up the healing process by repairing damaged tissues.

According to the Coconut Research Center, coconut kills viruses that cause influenza, measles, hepatitis, herpes, SARS, etc. It also kills bacteria that cause ulcers, throat infections, urinary tract infections, pneumonia, etc. In addition, it helps in controlling blood sugar and improves the secretion of insulin.

Ingestion of coconut oil occurs primarily through cooking oil. It helps improve the digestive system and thus prevents various stomach and digestion-related problems including irritable bowel syndrome. The saturated fats present in coconut oil have anti-microbial properties and help in dealing with various bacteria, parasites and fungi that cause indigestion. Coconut oil also helps in the absorption of other nutrients such as vitamins, minerals and amino acids.

Corn

Corn, alternatively called maize, is one of the most popular cereals in the world and forms the staple food in many countries. It not only provides the calories for daily metabolism but is a rich source of vitamins A, B, E and many minerals. Its high fibre content ensures that it plays a role in the prevention of digestive ailments like constipation and haemorrhoids as well as colorectal cancer. The antioxidants present in corn also act as anti-cancer agents and may help prevent Alzheimer's.

Being rich in phytochemicals, corn provides protection against numerous chronic diseases. It is rich in vitamin B nutrients, especially thiamine and niacin. Its consumption can provide a large chunk of the daily folate requirement and a rich source of beta-carotene which forms vitamin A in the body, essential for the maintenance of good vision and skin. Corn kernels are rich in vitamin E, a natural antioxidant essential for growth.

Corn also contains abundant phosphorus as well as magnesium, manganese, zinc, iron and copper. Phosphorus is essential for the maintenance of normal growth, bone health and normal kidney function. Magnesium is necessary for maintaining normal heart rate and for bone strength. Corn also contains trace minerals like selenium.

According to studies carried out at Cornell University, corn is a rich source of antioxidants, which fight the cancer-causing free radicals. It is a rich source of the phenolic compound ferulic acid, an anti-cancer agent which has been shown to be effective in fighting tumours in breast and liver cancers. The vitamin B12 and folic acid present in corn prevent anaemia caused by the deficiency of these vitamins.

Courgettes

Courgettes are an excellent source of manganese and vitamin C and a very good source of magnesium, vitamin A, fibre, potassium, folate, copper, riboflavin and phosphorus. High intake of fibre rich foods helps to keep cancer-causing toxins away from cells in the colon, while the folate, vitamin C and beta-carotene also have anti-inflammatory properties that make them helpful in combating conditions like asthma, osteoarthritis and rheumatoid arthritis.

The magnesium in courgettes has been shown to be helpful for reducing the risk of heart attack and stroke. Together with the potassium in courgettes, magnesium is also helpful in reducing high blood pressure. The vitamin C and beta-carotene can help to prevent the oxidation of cholesterol and the vitamin folate found in courgettes is needed by the body to break down a dangerous metabolic by-product called homocysteine, which can contribute to heart attack and stroke if levels get too high.

Courgettes have been found to have anti-cancer type effects. Although phytonutrient research on courgettes is limited, some lab studies have shown vegetable juices obtained from courgettes to be equivalent to juices made from leeks, and pumpkin in their ability to prevent cell mutations.

Cucumbers

Even though fresh cucumbers are mostly composed of water, they are packed full with nutrition. Cucumber flesh is a very good source of vitamins A and C and folic acid. The skin is rich in fibre and a variety of minerals including magnesium, molybdenum and potassium.

Cucumber skin is also an excellent source of silica, which is a trace mineral that contributes to the strength of our connective tissue, which is what holds our body together. Cucumbers are effective when used for various skin problems, including swelling under the eyes and sunburn. They also contain ascorbic and caffeic acids, which prevent water retention. That may explain why, when cucumbers are applied topically, they are often helpful for swollen eyes, burns and dermatitis.

Cucumbers' nutritional benefits include natural salts, enzymes and vitamins essential for strong cell growth and repair. In addition, the high mineral content and minerals in the skin offer a natural source for a fresh, powerful antioxidant. The cucumber is also a top choice as a diuretic. It can help control constipation, stomach disorders, arthritis, cholera and acne. The high water content, combined with its ability to balance acid, helps to reduce disorders and ailments that may be a cause of overproduction of various acidic compounds.

Dark Chocolate

Chocolate is made from plants, which means it contains many of the health benefits of dark vegetables. These benefits are from flavonoids, which act as antioxidants. Dark chocolate (more than 70% cocoa) contains a large number of antioxidants (nearly eight times the amount found in strawberries). Flavonoids also help relax blood pressure through the production of nitric oxide and balance certain hormones in the body. Dark chocolate is good for your heart. A small bar every day can help keep your heart and cardiovascular system running well, reduce blood pressure and LDL cholesterol by up to 10 percent.

A research study published by Joe A. Vinson of the University of Scranton, Pennsylvania, found that the flavonoids in dark chocolate are more powerful than vitamins such as ascorbic acid in protecting circulating lipids from oxidation in the blood stream and clogging the arteries. They also make blood platelets less likely to stick together and cause clots. Flavonoids are plant compounds with potent antioxidant properties; so far scientists have found more than 4,000 types. Cocoa beans contain large quantities of flavonoids, as do red wine, tea and cranberries.

The type of flavonoids found in chocolate are called flavonols. Generally, science has found that dark chocolate is higher in flavonoids than milk chocolate, as the way that cocoa powder and chocolate syrups are manufactured removes most flavonoids.

Fish

Although no single food alone can make a person healthy, eating more seafood is one way that most of us can help improve our diets and our health. Many of the studies about beneficial omega-3 fatty acids focus on fish as the primary source. Wild salmon, sardines, tuna and even shellfish are rich in omega-3 fatty acids and eating more of all types of fish and seafood is recommended.

The health benefits of fish oil include its ability to contribute to the prevention of heart disease, high cholesterol, depression, anxiety, cancer, diabetes, inflammation, etc. Most of the health benefits can be attributed to the presence of omega-3 essential fatty acids such as docosahexaenoic acid (DHA) and eicosapentaenoic acid (EPA). Other useful essential fatty acids include alpha-linolenic acid (ALA) and gamma-linolenic acid (GLA).

The various types of fish which can be a good source of fish oil are mackerel, rainbow trout, lake trout, halibut, herring, sea bass, sardines, swordfish, oysters, albacore tuna, blue fin tuna, yellow fin tuna, turbot, pilchards, anchovies and wild salmon. The most common among these for obtaining fish oil are albacore tuna, herring, mackerel, sardines, lake trout and wild salmon.

Hundreds of studies have been done on fish or fish oils and their role in the prevention or treatment of heart disease. A review in the *British Medical Journal* recommends fish or fish oil supplements to prevent heart attacks, particularly in people with vascular disease. How omega-3 fat reduces heart disease is not known, but they are known to lower blood triglycerides and blood pressure, prevent clotting, they are anti-inflammatory and reduce abnormal heart rhythms.

Flaxseed

Consuming flaxseed is associated with a reduction in total cholesterol, including the LDL ('bad') cholesterol and triglycerides. Study after study has shown a positive response to eating ground flaxseed daily. Eating low fat foods, increasing exercise, limiting salt and sugar, and eating flaxseed daily are a few ways that you can win the battle against high cholesterol.

Flaxseed is high in lignans, up to 800 times the amount found in any other tested plant food. Lignans, a phytoestrogen, have been called by H. Adlercreutz (in his article 'Phytoestrogens: Epidemology and a Possible Role in Cancer Prevention') natural cancer-protective compounds. Flaxseed is also high in alpha-linolenic acid (ALA), which has been found to be a promising cancer fighting agent. The American National Cancer Institute has singled out flaxseed as one of six foods that deserve special study. Flaxseed's high fibre aspect is also beneficial in the fight against colon cancer. Epidemiological studies note that diet plays a major role in the incidence of colon cancer. Research has shown that increasing the amount of fibre in your diet reduces breast and colon cancer risk. It is thought that lignan metabolites can bind to oestrogen receptors, thereby inhibiting the onset of oestrogen-stimulated breast cancer.

Goji Berries

Goji berries are rich in antioxidants, particularly carotenoids such as beta-carotene and zeaxanthin. Exposure to chemicals, pollutants and free radicals can cause DNA damage and breakage, leading to genetic mutations, cancer, etc. Gojis' betaine and master molecule polysaccharides can restore and repair damaged DNA.

Goji were shown to enhance the effect of radiation in combating lung cancer, allowing a lower dose to be used. Other research indicates that goji can protect against some of the nauseous side effects of chemotherapy and radiation. It was also found that goji can reduce the time it takes for vision to adapt to darkness. The carotenoids in goji may protect against macular degeneration and cataracts.

Some scientists believe that goji may be an especially good supplement to prevent liver cancer because it provides protection against liver damage and anti-cancer effects at the same time. Goji is believed to have the potential to diminish tumour cells by inducing apoptosis, a process in which cancer cells are broken down and recycled.

Goji is considered to be 'brain tonic' because of its betaine content, which is converted in the body into choline. These are substances that enhance memory and recall ability. Goji can help to strengthen your immune system and heart, help support normal kidney and liver function, maintain a healthy cholesterol level, normalize blood pressure, prevent and control diabetes. It can also help to strengthen the muscles and bones, maintain healthy gums, improve your digestion, and help you get a good night's sleep. Who knew that a tiny fruit could pack so many benefits?

Green Peas

Green peas provide high amounts of vitamins, minerals, dietary fibre and protein. They are a very good source of vitamin K, some of which our bodies convert into K2, which activates osteocalcin, the major non-collagen protein in the bone. Osteocalcin anchors calcium molecules inside the bone; without enough vitamin K2, osteocalcin levels are inadequate and bone mineralization is impaired.

Green peas also serve as a very good source of folic acid and vitamin B6. These two nutrients help to reduce the build up of homocysteine, a dangerous molecule which can obstruct collagen cross-linking, resulting in poor bone matrix and osteoporosis. One study showed that by supplementing with folic acid, post menopausal women who were not considered deficient in folic acid lowered their homocysteine levels.

Green Tea

The secret of green tea lies in the fact that it is rich in polyphenols, particularly epigallocatechin gallate (EGCG). EGCG is a powerful antioxidant. Besides inhibiting the growth of cancer cells, it kills them without harming healthy tissue. It has also been effective in lowering LDL ('bad') cholesterol levels, and inhibiting the abnormal formation of blood clots. The latter takes on added importance when you consider that thrombosis (the formation of blood clots) is the leading cause of heart attacks and strokes.

Green, oolong and black teas all come from the leaves of the Camellia Sinensis plant. What sets green tea apart is the way it is processed. Green tea leaves are steamed, which prevents the EGCG compound from being oxidized. By contrast, black and oolong tea leaves are made from fermented leaves, which results in the EGCG being converted into other compounds that are not nearly as effective in preventing and fighting various diseases.

Hazelnuts

Hazelnuts are a very important food item in a well-balanced diet. They provide several important health benefits in protecting against diseases. Hazelnuts and hazelnut oil are the best known sources of vitamin E, which is essential for healthy heart muscles and other muscles of the body. It is also necessary for normal functioning of the reproductive system. Vitamin E prevents the disintegration of red blood cells, and so serves as protection against anaemia. Hazelnuts are a useful source of thiamine, which enhances and promotes normal appetite, and vitamin B6 which aids protein metabolism and absorption.

Hazelnuts are also good sources of protein, dietary fibre, iron, calcium and potassium. Although high in fat, they contain no cholesterol. Like other varieties of nuts, hazelnuts also contain significant amounts of phytochemicals, which have antioxidant properties that protect the body against several types of cancer.

Kale

Kale is a leafy green vegetable with a mild earthy flavour. The season for kale is between mid winter and early spring. It is rich in calcium, lutein, iron and vitamins A and K. It has seven times the beta-carotene of broccoli and ten times more lutein. Kale is rich in vitamins C, E and fibre. Kale's important attributes are the natural occurring all important phytochemicals sulforaphane and indoles which research suggests may protect against cancer.

Science has discovered that sulforaphane helps boost the body's detoxification enzymes, possibly by altering gene expression. This in turn is purported to help clear carcinogenic substances in a timely manner. Sulforaphane is formed when cruciferous vegetables like kale and cabbage are chopped or chewed. This somehow triggers the liver to produce enzymes that detoxify cancer-causing chemicals, to which we are all exposed to on a daily basis. A study in the *Journal of Nutrition* (2004) demonstrates that sulforaphane helps stop breast cancer cell proliferation.

Kiwi fruit

Kiwi fruit are rich in many vitamins, flavonoids and minerals. In particular, they contain a high amount of vitamin C (more than oranges), as much potassium as bananas and a good amount of beta-carotene. It is also important to note that kiwi fruit contain a remarkable amount of vitamins E and A.

Vitamin C is a water-soluble antioxidant that has been proven to protect our body from free radicals, dramatically improving the health of those who consume it regularly against all kinds of diseases, from cardiovascular problems to cancer and obesity. Vitamin E has been proven to have similar effects, but it is fat-soluble and therefore complementary to the functions of vitamin C. Kiwi fruit contain both these vitamins in high amounts, helping to protect our body from free radicals from all fronts.

The high content of dietary fibre helps improve diseases such as diabetes and colon cancer by controlling sugar levels, since fibre binds to toxic compounds in the colon and helps us expel them.

Leeks

Leeks have similar nutritional benefits to onions and garlic. They provide a good source of fibre, folic acid, vitamins B6 and C, manganese and iron. As leeks are less dense than onions and garlic, larger quantities of them need to be consumed in order to produce similar beneficial effects.

Studies have shown that leeks can improve the immune system, lower bad cholesterol levels and fight cancer. Modern researchers have found leeks, as well as most of the plants in the onion family, to be highly beneficial when consumed in moderation (two to seven times a week). They have been shown to reduce bad cholesterol and raise good cholesterol levels in the body. They will also help keep down high blood pressure.

Leeks are believed to fight cancer, especially colon and prostate cancer. They contain quercetin and other compounds which inhibit carcinogenic development and also restrict the spread of cancer. Leeks also contain kaempferol, a substance which has been shown to reduce ovarian cancer in women. The green parts of leeks are especially nutritious as they contain B vitamins and are loaded with protective antioxidants such as carotenoids, lutein, and zeaxanthin.

Lentils

Lentils are a small but nutritionally mighty member of the legume family and also a very good source of cholesterol-lowering fibre because of their soluble fibre content. They are beneficial in managing blood sugar disorders since their high fibre content prevents blood sugar levels from rising rapidly after a meal. Lentils are very rich in protein, folic acid, and vitamins C and B. They also contain eight of the essential amino acids, thereby providing a great dietary source to vegetarians.

There is evidence to prove that lentils can slow the liver's manufacture of cholesterol, which similarly helps to reduce levels in the body. A study carried out by the Department of Nutrition at the Harvard School of Public Health, Boston, has shown that women with diets high in lentils and peas (which both contain high levels of flavones) have a reduced risk of breast cancer. The intake of dietary fibre, particularly from lentils, has also been known to reduce the risk of coronary heart disease.

Lentils are relatively quick and easy to prepare. They readily absorb a variety of wonderful flavours from other foods and seasonings, are high in nutritional value and are available throughout the year.

Miso

Miso is made of soya beans and koji, a culture starter made from beneficial moulds, yeast and lactic acid bacteria. Making miso is an art form in Japan. As long as you choose unpasteurized miso, you will be getting the benefits of live, friendly microflora for a healthy digestive system. There are many types of miso, some made with just soya beans and soya koji (called hatcho miso, a favourite in Japan) and others made with barley and rice. Miso soup is rich in antioxidants and protective fatty acids, and a healthy dose of vitamin E. It also contains protein and vitamin B12, and a good selection of minerals to help boost your immune system.

Miso soup is said to help regulate the oestrogen hormone in women, a hormone that can cause tumours to develop. Many studies have been done on miso, some on humans and some on animals. These studies show that it helps reduce the risk of cancers like breast, prostate, lung and colon cancers. Miso provides protein, vitamins B2, E and K, tryptophan, choline, dietary fibre, linoleic acid and lecithin, which help maintain nutritional balance and preserve healthy skin. The isoflavones in miso have been shown to reduce menopausal symptoms like hot flushes.

Mushrooms

Mushrooms are an excellent source of potassium, a mineral that helps lower elevated blood pressure and reduces the risk of stroke. One medium portobello mushroom has even more potassium than a banana or a glass of orange juice. One serving of mushrooms provides about 20 to 40 percent of the daily value of copper which has cardio-protective properties.

Mushrooms are a rich source of riboflavin, niacin and selenium. Selenium is an antioxidant that works with vitamin E to protect cells from damaging effects of free radicals. In one study, male health professionals who consumed twice the recommended daily intake of selenium cut their risk of prostate cancer by 65 percent.

Like most plants, mushrooms are loaded with polysaccharides, phytonutrients that appear to possess potent anti-cancer properties. Several studies indicate that mushrooms may help to prevent breast cancer. This is attributed to the inhibition of aromatase, an enzyme involved in hyperestrogenemia, a condition characterized by excessive oestrogen production. Mushrooms are also high in other antioxidants such as L-ergothioneine. In fact, they contain higher levels of this agent than other dietary sources, including liver and wheat germ, and are not depleted during cooking.

According to the *Journal of Neurology, Neurosurgery & Psychiatry*, the prevention of Alzheimer's disease may be included among the health benefits of mushrooms. This assessment is based on research suggesting that niacin-rich foods, like mushrooms, appear to prevent or delay Alzheimer's and other cognitive disorders by as much as 70 percent. In addition, niacin interrupts the activity of homocysteine, an amino acid associated with elevated cholesterol and an increased risk of heart disease, stroke and osteoarthritis.

Mushrooms are an excellent source of iron, selenium, potassium, phosphorus, riboflavin, pantothenis acid, copper and zinc. In addition to providing antioxidant value, these nutrients also play a role in enhancing immunity and preventing disease. Most of the research completed on the health benefits of mushrooms has focused on the shiitake, maitake, reishi and crimini varieties. More recent research indicates that common white button mushrooms provide just as much potential to fight cancer and reduce blood pressure and cholesterol as fancier varieties. This includes portobello mushrooms, the popular vegetarian meat alternative. Oyster and thistle mushrooms contain about 80 to 90 percent water, and are very low in calories. They have little sodium and fat, and 8 to 10 percent of the dry weight is fibre.

Olives

Even though olives have a high fat content of 15 to 35 percent, they are an excellent source of oleic acid (an omega-9 monounsaturated fatty acid). Since olives contain mixed tocopherols, they are also a good source of vitamin E. Olives and their oil contain many unique phenolic and aromatic compounds, including oleuroperin and flavonoids.

Research has shown that it is the type of fat consumed that determines the risk of developing conditions such as diabetes, atherosclerosis, colon cancer, arthritis and asthma. People from regions such as the Mediterranean typically consume large amounts of olive oil and have a lower risk of developing those conditions.

In places like the United States, high levels of animal fats are consumed which increases the risk of developing those diseases. Olives and olive oil may also be effective in the prevention and treatment of asthma, cancer and arthritis.

Onions

Onions are a surprising source of fibre and a rich source of healthy sulphur compounds, similar to those found in garlic. Research on onions appears to have lagged behind garlic research, but onions seem to have similar cardiovascular benefits, such as reducing blood pressure and blood cholesterol levels, at least in the short term. Onions have antibacterial and antifungal properties, and also contain flavonoids, which help vitamin C in its function, improving the integrity of blood vessels and decreasing inflammation.

Onions also contain vitamin C and chromium. Chromium is a mineral that helps cells respond to insulin, ultimately assisting with blood glucose control. Green onions, because of their bright green tops, provide a wealth of vitamin A. Onions are a very good source of vitamin B6, biotin and fibre. They are also a good source of folic acid and vitamins B1 and K.

The health benefits provided by onions are mostly due to the several organic sulphur compounds they contain. Like garlic, onions also have the enzyme allinase (released when an onion is cut or crushed). Other constituents that are found in onions include phenolic acids (such as ellagic, caffeic, sinapic and p-coumaric), pectin, sterols, saponins and volatile oils.

Pears

Pears are an excellent source of soluble fibre. They contain vitamins A, B1, B2, C, E, folic acid and niacin. They are also rich in copper, phosphorus and potassium, with lesser amounts of calcium, chlorine, iron, magnesium, sodium and sulphur. Some varieties have more iron content than others.

Pears have antioxidant and anti-carcinogen glutathione, which help prevent high blood pressure and stroke. The high vitamin C and copper content act as good antioxidants that protect cells from damage by free radicals and are critical in building the immune system. The high content of pectin in pears makes this fruit very useful in lowering cholesterol levels. The pectin is also a diuretic and has a mild laxative effect. Drinking pear juice regularly helps regulate bowel movements. Due to its high amount of fructose and glucose, pear juice is a quick and natural source of energy. It is also high in fibre, which is highly beneficial for colon health. Pear juice has an anti-inflammatory effect and helps relieve sufferers of much pain in various inflammatory conditions. Pears also contain high levels of boron, which assists in retaining calcium and thus prevents or stops osteoporosis.

Peppers

Brightly coloured bell peppers, whether green, red, orange or yellow, are rich sources of some of the best nutrients available. Peppers are an excellent source of vitamins C and A, two very powerful antioxidants. These antioxidants work together to effectively neutralize free radicals, which can travel through the body causing huge amounts of damage to cells which can lead to heart disease, cataracts, asthma, diabetes, etc. By providing these two potent free radical destroyers, bell peppers may help prevent or reduce some of the symptoms of these conditions by shutting down the source of the problem.

As mentioned above, all peppers are rich in vitamins A, C and K, but red peppers are simply bursting with them. Vitamins A and C also reduce inflammation like that found in arthritis and asthma. Vitamin K promotes proper blood clotting, strengthens bones and helps protect cells from oxidative damage.

Red peppers are a good source of the carotenoid called lycopene, an antioxidant compound that is earning a reputation for helping prevent prostate cancer as well as cancer of the bladder, cervix and pancreas. Beta-cryptoxanthin, another carotenoid in red peppers, helps to prevent lung cancer related to smoking and second-hand smoke. Besides being rich in phytochemicals, peppers provide a decent amount of fibre.

Pineapples

Pineapple is packed full of vitamins and minerals. Its nutrients include calcium, potassium, fibre and vitamin C. In addition, it is low in fat and cholesterol. Pineapple also contains a substance called bromelain, which is a natural anti-inflammatory that has many health benefits and encourages healing. According to Dr Andrew Weil, bromelain is very effective in treating bruises, sprains and strains by reducing swelling, tenderness and pain. This powerful anti-inflammatory effect can also help relieve rheumatoid arthritis symptoms and reduce post-operative swelling. Additionally, the bromelain contained in fresh pineapple can relieve indigestion. This enzyme breaks down the amino acid bonds in proteins which promotes good digestion.

Pineapples provide an ample supply of vitamin C, a commonly known antioxidant (as previously mentioned) that protects the body from free radical damage and boosts the immune system.

Pomegranates

Pomegranate contains polyphenols, tannins and anthocyanins, all of which are beneficial antioxidants. Its high antioxidant content rivals that of many other fruits, red wine and green tea.

Pomegranate juice also contains fibre, potassium and vitamin C. Studies are being carried out to research the health benefits of pomegranate juice in possibly decreasing the return rate of prostate cancer after surgery and chemotherapy. It may also prevent hardening of the arteries by keeping the arteries clear from fatty deposits and may even slow the progression of heart disease.

The antioxidant properties of pomegranate help to guard the body against the substances that can cause premature aging, heart disease, Alzheimer's, cancer and other diseases or conditions. It has been used around the world as a way to clear skin. In folk medicine it has been used to treat inflammation, sore throats and rheumatism.

Quinoa

Quinoa (pronounced keen-wah) is not a grain; it is actually a seed of a plant which belongs to the spinach family. When cooked, quinoa is light and fluffy, slightly crunchy and subtly flavoured. It in fact cooks and tastes like a grain, making it an excellent replacement for grains that are difficult to digest or that feed candida (a systemic fungal infection).

Researchers attribute the health benefits of quinoa to its complete nutritional makeup. Quinoa is close to being one of the most complete foods in nature because it contains amino acids, enzymes, vitamins and minerals, fibre, antioxidants and phytonutrients. Quinoa contains all nine essential amino acids that are required by the body as building blocks for muscles. It also contains high levels of magnesium, which helps to relax the muscles and blood vessels, which in turn lowers blood pressure.

Quinoa is a wonderful way to ensure that you consume valuable fibre that eases elimination and tones your colon. It is also a good source of manganese and copper which act as antioxidants in the body to get rid of dangerous cancer and disease-causing substances. Studies have shown that in its whole grain form, quinoa may be effective in preventing and treating artherosclerosis, breast cancer, diabetes and insulin resistance.

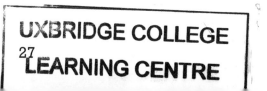

Raisins

Raisins are used worldwide in cuisines (especially desserts), health tonics and as snacks. They are made from drying grapes (green or black), either in the sun or in driers and they look like golden, green or black gems.

Raisins contain vitamin B, which is known for boosting energy. They are also high in calories, which is important for athletes as it helps boost energy naturally.

They help relieve constipation, anaemia, fever, and help in weight gain, eye care, dental care and bone health. The juice of soaked or stewed raisins has been found to be a good remedy for sore throat, asthma and cases of cold. Raisins contain oleic acid, which helps promote good oral health by destroying the bacteria that cause cavities. They are also rich in iron, fibre and tartaric which promote digestive health and regularity. Research has found that eating two servings a day may help lower the risk of colon cancer. They are one of the best dietary sources of boron, which is essential for bone health. The minerals in raisins in conjunction with oestrogen in women help make bones stronger and ward off osteoporosis.

Raisins are rich in antioxidants that help protect our bodies against free radical damage. They can help lower cholesterol and reduce the risk of heart disease. The fruit sugar in raisins is more digestible than cane sugar and will not wreck havoc with blood sugar levels.

Red Wine

Recent studies show that drinking one glass of red wine each day may have certain health benefits. Research also indicates that moderate red wine consumption may help protect against certain cancers and heart disease, and can have a positive effect on cholesterol levels and blood pressure. The key to reaping the health benefits seems to be moderate consumption, so don't think that by drinking a bottle you would be getting these benefits – it doesn't work that way! Drinking one glass a day for women and up to two glasses a day for men may reduce the risk of heart disease, cancer or stroke.

The compounds found in red wine that are responsible for its healing powers are antioxidants. Red wine contains several antioxidants beneficial to good health. One of the most studied antioxidants is resveratrol, a compound found in the seeds and skins of grapes. Red wine has a high concentration of resveratrol because the skins and seeds ferment in the grape juices during the wine-making process. This prolonged contact during fermentation produces significant levels of resveratrol in the finished red wine. White wine also contains resveratrol, but the seeds and skins are removed early in the wine making process, reducing the concentration of the compound in the finished white wine.

Found in red wine, peanuts, blueberries and cranberries, resveratrol is easily absorbed by the body. Its antioxidant properties also offer health benefits in the prevention of heart disease and the reduction of lung tissue inflammation in chronic obstructive pulmonary disease (COPD).

Studies have shown that resveratrol has the ability to inhibit the process that leads to the growth and spreading (metastasis) of cancer. Resveratrol helps to neutralize the oxidation of free radicals, which keeps them from penetrating the cell membrane and destroying the protein and DNA inside healthy cells. Resveratrol also shows properties of tumour suppression by preventing the production of new blood vessels, which can help limit the growth of tumours by cutting off their supply of nutrients.

Red wine also contains other antioxidants such as a flavonoid known as catechin, which is also present in green tea. Research indicates that along with resveratrol, catechin plays an important role in reducing the risk of heart disease. Saponins, also found in red wine, olive oil and soya beans, offer protective benefits for the heart and are easily absorbed by the body. Yet another antioxidant found in red wine, guercetin, is being studied for its value in the prevention of lung cancer.

Seaweed

As a food, seaweed is primarily used in certain salads, sushi and other ethnic oriented cuisines around the world, but food is not the only way to enjoy the benefits of seaweed. Studies show a vast array of overwhelming health benefits. Not only does seaweed have a wonderful effect on the thyroid because it normalizes and stabilizes its function but the benefits continue. It can also stabilize blood pressure, lower cholesterol and promote a healthy intestinal tract. The best nutritional benefit is, however, that various cancers among those who regularly consume seaweed are extremely low.

Seaweeds are algae and have unique health and nutritional properties. A list of some of the main types of seaweed and their main health benefits follows.

- Nori is rich in iodine and iron, and quite high in protein. It is also a good source of vitamins C and A, potassium, magnesium and riboflavin (B2), and it is low in fat.

- Dulse is exceptionally nutritious, containing around 10 to 20 percent protein and a whole host of vitamins and minerals, including magnesium, iron and beta-carotene (which the body uses to produce vitamin A). It is now being farmed in Ireland for its health benefits and for making skin care and cosmetic products.
- Carrageen or Irish moss (chondrus cripus) is widely used in all sorts of food products because it has emulsifying and gelling properties. It is used to thicken foods and produces a colourless jelly-like consistency, so it is used in lots of commercial desserts. It is also a vegetarian answer to gelatine. It was traditionally rated in Ireland as a cold and cough remedy. It is rich in retinol and minerals.
- Wakame is a green seaweed with a slippery consistency and an almost sweet taste. It has a thick band of fibre in the centre which can be easily cut out to give a more palatable effect. It can easily be added in small amounts to lots of cooked dishes such as stir-fries and stews, and is also delicious as a side dish. The Japanese use it as part of miso soup.
- Kelp (laminaria digitata) is found in many areas of the world. It is a brown seaweed with literally thousands of varieties. It is found in all sorts of com- mercial products, from toothpaste to fertilizer. As it is exceptionally rich in iodine, it used to be the main source for preventing goitre and treating thyroid conditions. It is still highly rated by naturopaths and nutritional therapists for that use.

Spinach

Spinach is one of the most beneficial and healthy vegetables, and is known to be a powerhouse of nutrients among all green leafy vegetables. It is filled with vitamins, proteins, antioxidants and essential nutrients that promote overall good health and well-being. To get the maximum health benefits from spinach, it should be consumed as soon as it is purchased. The longer it is refrigerated, the fewer nutrients it contains. When kept in the fridge for more than a week, fresh spinach tends to lose almost half its nutrients, so it's best to consume it in the shortest possible time.

Spinach and other dark leafy greens like kale, collard greens, Swiss chard, turnip greens and bok choy are loaded with calcium, folic acid, vitamin K and iron. Spinach is also rich in vitamin C, fibre and carotenoids. Include its lutein and bioflavonoid compounds, and spinach is a nutritional powerhouse. The calcium content strengthens bones, while the A and C vitamins plus fibre, folic acid, magnesium and other nutrients help control cancer, especially colon, lung and breast cancers. Folate also lowers the blood levels of homocysteine, which helps protect against heart disease.

The flavonoids in spinach help protect against age-related memory loss. Its secret weapon is lutein, which makes it one of the best foods in the world to prevent cataracts, as well as age-related macular degeneration, the leading cause of preventable blindness in the elderly. Foods rich in lutein are also thought to help prevent cancer.

Sweet Potatoes

Sweet potatoes provide an excellent source of carotenes and the darker varieties contain a higher concentration. They also offer a good source of vitamins B2, B6 and C, manganese, copper, biotin, pantothenic acid and fibre. Sweet potatoes contain unique root storage proteins, which have been shown to have significant antioxidant effects. Being rich in dietary fibre, they lower the risk of constipation, diverticulosis, colon and rectal cancer.

Sweet potatoes have been found to be helpful in minimizing the risk of heart disease, diabetes and obesity. Eating sweet potatoes has been known to help in avoiding stroke, by bringing down the harmful effects of low-density cholesterol and preventing blood clots.

The presence of beta-carotene in sweet potatoes helps the body fight against free radicals and thus assists in preventing cancer. Since they have a low glycemic index (GI), they can be consumed by those suffering from diabetes without concern. The high amount of potassium helps the body in maintaining fluid and electrolyte balance as well as cell integrity.

Sweet potatoes have been found to be beneficial for blood purification as well as lowering of blood pressure. Owing to the presence of calcium and iron, they ensure proper blood flow and also improve bone density. Regular consumption of sweet potato is good for stomach ulcers and inflamed condition of the colon.

Swiss Chard

Swiss chard is a tall, leafy green vegetable with a thick, crunchy stalk that comes in white, red or yellow with wide fan-like green leaves. Chard belongs to the same family as beets and spinach, and shares a similar taste profile. Both the leaves and stalk are edible, although the stems vary in texture with the white ones being the most tender.

The leaves and roots have been the subject of fascinating health studies. The combination of traditional nutrients, phytonutrients (particularly anthocyans) plus fibre seems particularly effective in preventing digestive tract cancers. Several research studies on chard focus specifically on colon cancer, where the incidence of precancerous lesions in animals has been found to be significantly reduced following dietary intake of swiss chard extracts or fibre.

Swiss chard is also a very good source of copper, calcium, vitamins B1, B2 and B6, protein, phosphorus, zinc, folate, biotin, niacin and pantothenic acid.

Tamarind

Tamarind is a long bean-like pod that belongs to the vegetable order but is treated like a fruit. Its name is derived from the Arabic word 'tamar', meaning a dry date fruit. It was the Arabs in India who gave the name of 'tamar-hindi' to this tree.

Tamarind is green when immature and, when it matures, it becomes fatter and changes colour to a sandy brown. Its flesh consists of dry, sticky, dark brown pulp and inside the pulp are shiny black seeds. It is this pulp that people eat to get all the nutritional and health benefits of the tamarind. The pulp has a very sour taste while it is young. As it ripens it gets sweeter, although the tamarind generally has a sour, acidic taste which is a favourite flavouring for a host of fish and curry dishes.

The pulp is used for jams, syrups and sweets. In the west, tamarind is used in the preparation of Worcestershire and barbecue sauces, and other meat condiments.

Tamarind is a good source of antioxidants that fight against cancer. It contains carotenes, vitamins C and B, and flavonoids. Tamarind lowers cholesterol and promotes a healthy heart.

Tofu

Tofu is a low-fat, low-cholesterol, low-calorie food made from steamed and compressed soya beans. Not only is it a great source of protein, which many vegetarians lack, but it is also heart-healthy and has been linked to a decreased risk in cancer. In addition to being used as a meat alternative, tofu is served in a number of spicy and ethnic dishes, which were never intended to contain meat. Many ethnic Indian dishes contain large amounts of tofu, cooked and spiced in different ways.

Tofu is rich in both high quality protein and B vitamins making it an excellent substitute for meat in many vegetarian recipes. It contains a lot of calcium, which originates from the coagulant (nigari). When making tofu, the soya proteins are precipitated with calcium, providing a ready source of calcium, which contributes to the prevention of osteoporosis.

An additional benefit is that tofu is extremely easy to digest. This is because the soya bean's fibre is removed during the manufacturing process. As with most other soya foods, tofu reduces heart disease by lowering the level of LDL ('bad') cholesterol and, as a result, maintaining the level of good cholesterol (HDL).

Tofu is rich in isoflavones. During the manufacture of tofu, the soya isoflavones, genistein and daidzein, remain bound to the soya protein. Firm tofu contains about 35 mg of isoflavones per 100g. Isoflavones reduce the risk of osteoporosis, lower rates of breast and prostate cancers, and reduce menopausal symptoms including mood swings and hot flushes.

Tomatoes

Tomatoes, which are actually a fruit and not a vegetable, are loaded with all kinds of health benefits for the body. They are in fact a highly-versatile health product and, due to their equally versatile preparation options, there's really no reason to neglect them as part of a healthy diet.

One of the best-known benefits of the tomato is its lycopene content. Lycopene is a vital antioxidant that helps in the fight against cancerous cell formation as well as other types of health complications and diseases. Free radicals in the body are neutralized by the high levels of lycopene, and the tomato is so amply loaded with this vital antioxidant from which it actually derives its rich redness.

Lycopene is not produced within the human body so we require sources of lycopene in order to make use of this powerful antioxidant. While other fruits and vegetables contain necessary health ingredients, none have the tomato's high concentration of lycopene. Cancers such as prostate, cervical, colon, rectal, and cancers of the stomach, mouth, pharynx and oesophagus have all been proven to be staved off by high levels of lycopene. Researchers introduced lycopene into pre-existing cancer cell cultures and it prevented the continued growth of these cultures. This is pretty powerful evidence that the health-benefits of eating tomatoes are really quite phenomenal.

When choosing your tomatoes, be sure to pick those with the most brilliant shades of red, which indicate the highest amounts of beta-carotene and lycopene. Though raw tomatoes are very good for you, cooking them releases even more benefits. Lycopene is located in the cell wall of the tomato so by cooking in a little olive oil this healing compound is more fully released, allowing your body to absorb it better. Tomatoes do not lose any of their nutritional value in high-heat processing, making canned tomatoes and tomato sauce just as viable and beneficial as fresh tomatoes.

Turkey

Turkey is a very good source of protein, selenium, niacin, vitamins B6 and B12, zinc and the amino acid tryptophan. The skinless white meat is an excellent high-protein, low-fat food. It also has less saturated fat, less total fat and less cholesterol than chicken, pork or beef.

The health benefits of turkey include reducing LDL ('bad') cholesterol, mood-enhancing properties, helping to prevent cancer, boosting testosterone and the immune system. The amino acid tryptophan is needed for T cells, a type of immune system cell that kills cancer cells. T cells activated in the absence of free tryptophan become susceptible to death via apoptosis. Neurotransmitters are made from amino acids, and the neurotransmitter serotonin is made from tryptophan. Serotonin helps to improve mood and eating food such as turkey can help improve your mood.

Turkey contains selenium, which plays an essential role in helping to eliminate cancer-friendly free radicals in the body. It is a good source of vitamins B3 and B6. Vitamin B3 helps lower blood cholesterol, is essential for healthy skin and helps improve brain function. Vitamin B6 helps in maintaining muscle tone, aids in the production of anti-bodies and red blood cells and is essential for normal growth. A serving of turkey meat has 36 percent of the daily allowance of vitamin B3 and 27 percent of your recommended daily intake of vitamin B6. Without the skin turkey is naturally low in fat; it only contains 1g of fat per 28g of flesh.

Walnuts

Walnuts are one of the best plant sources of protein. They are rich in fibre, B vitamins, magnesium and antioxidants such as vitamin E. Nuts in general are also high in plant sterols and fat, but mostly monounsaturated and polyunsaturated fats (omega-3 fatty acids – the good fats) that have been shown to lower LDL ('bad') cholesterol. Walnuts, in particular, have significantly higher amounts of omega-3 fatty acids as compared to other nuts.

Walnuts have also been shown to aid in lowering the C-reactive protein (CRP) level in the blood. CRP was recently recognized as an independent marker and predictor of heart disease. They are a very good source of manganese and copper, two minerals that are essential co-factors in a number of enzymes important in antioxidant defences. Walnuts also contain an antioxidant compound called ellagic acid, which not only helps protect healthy cells from free radical damage but also helps detoxify potential cancer-causing substances helping to prevent cancer cells from replicating.

Yams

Yams provide a very good source of potassium and fibre. They also offer a good source of vitamins B1, B6 and C, manganese and carbohydrates. Yams contain a unique phytoestrogen called diosgenin that is used as a starting material for the synthesis of the hormones oestrogen and progesterone which is created by drug manufacturers. Yams are a superfood, especially as they possess phytoestrogen activity. They contain large amounts of vitamin B6, which is required by the liver, and also contain folic acid and other B vitamins, which help to detoxify excess oestrogen.

Yams' complex carbohydrates and fibre deliver the goods, gradually, slowing the rate at which their sugars are released and absorbed into the bloodstream. In addition, because they are rich in fibre, yams fill you up without filling out your waistline. They are a good source of manganese, a trace mineral that helps with carbohydrate metabolism and a co-factor in a number of enzymes important in energy production and antioxidant defences.

Yams are a good source of potassium and vitamin B6, which are needed by the body to help control blood pressure and to break down homocysteine which can directly damage blood vessel walls. Since high homocysteine levels are significantly associated with increased risk of heart attack and stroke, having a good supply of vitamin B6 on hand makes a great deal of sense.

Yellow Split Peas

Of all legumes, yellow split peas have the most genistein, an isoflavone that research shows may help reduce your chances of heart disease. According to dietician Laurie Mozian, they provide nearly twice as much genistein as soya beans. Additionally, genistein binds to oestrogen receptors in your body, which may lower circulating oestrogen, a risk factor for breast cancer.

Split peas, a small but nutritionally mighty member of the legume family, are a very good source of cholesterol-lowering fibre. They are also of special benefit in managing blood sugar disorders since their high fibre content prevents blood sugar levels from rising rapidly after a meal. Studies have shown that type 2 diabetics who eat at least 50g of fibre a day can lower considerably their cholesterol, triglycerides and LDL (low density lipoprotein).

Dried peas also provide good to excellent amounts of minerals, B-vitamins and protein, and are virtually fat free. Yellow split peas have an earthy flavour with a creamy texture. Peas can also reduce the amount of plaque in your blood vessels and help your heart remain healthy.

Split peas come in two varieties: green and yellow. Both can be used for most recipes interchangeably. The most common way is split pea soup, which can be made with leftover meat or kept vegetarian. Split peas can also be made into a dip and enjoyed with pitta bread in the same way as hummus (see the recipe in Chapter 8).

Indian cuisine uses a lot of yellow split peas, in the form of daal. They are added to soups or used to make fava, which is a purée served with fish, salty foods or dark leafy greens. Split peas are also added to buckwheat or quinoa dishes in Indian cooking.

Yoghurt

Yoghurt provides a cooling contrast to the hotter, spicier Indian dishes, and is often served as a side dish, with salad or lassi, a popular yoghurt-based beverage that comes in flavours like mango, rose-water or salted.

Traditionally, yoghurt is a fermented dairy product made by adding bacteria to milk. The good bacteria in yoghurt (provided it is still live, which is not the case in many pasteurized varieties) has been found to enhance the immune system, improve arthritis, fight stomach ulcers and promote good digestion. Yoghurt is also a good source of calcium and has been found to promote fat loss while retaining lean muscles.

This fermented milk product has been around for thousands of years. In fact, it is believed that it originated in Bulgaria. From the Gaelic people to the Mongolians, yoghurt is a staple food for many traditional cultures. These cultures had no heart disease and lived on diets of mainly fermented milk products and meats. The key was that their milk was raw, not pasteurized. Pasteurization destroys many helpful enzymes in the yoghurt and other cultured milk products.
Yoghurt can also decrease your risk of contracting colon cancer because it contains lacto bacteria. Lacto bacteria is 'good bacteria' because it helps to keep your colon clean and free of wastes, while aiding digestion. Yoghurt is also a rich source of calcium, as most dairy products are. Eating it on a daily basis can help you absorb the nutrients, such as calcium and B vitamins, in other foods more readily, so you get the most nutritional value out of your meals. It can also boost your immune system, making your body better equipped to fight off toxins.

Chapter 2

Oils

There are many types of oils on the market, good and bad. I have chosen to list those which I use because of their content and health benefits. There are a lot of other healthy oils available which have very useful benefits, but there's only so much oil you can use.

The smoke point refers to the temperature at which cooking oil begins to break down, marking the point at which you start to lose the flavour and nutritional value.

Avocado Oil

Avocado oil is pressed and extracted from either the fresh flesh or dried pulp of avocados. The best culinary grade avocado oil is produced by cold pressing the oil from the fresh flesh of avocados, in a manner similar to the production of cold-pressed olive oil. Avocado oil can also be extracted from the dehydrated pulp of avocados, either through pressing or chemical/solvent extraction (which is typically employed for the avocado oil used as a base in cosmetics).

Avocado oil typically comes in one of two forms: refined or unrefined. Refined avocado oil has a lighter colour and a milder flavour with a very high smoke point that makes it ideal not only for salads, but especially for light frying and sautéing. The unrefined version of avocado oil is cloudier, has a deeper green colour and a deeper, more intense avocado flavour. Because unrefined avocado oils have more solids in them, they also have lower smoke points than refined avocado oils. This makes them ideal for salad dressings where a more intense flavour is desired or for other uses that don't involve heating the oil such as in dips for bread or finishing oil for vegetables.

Like olive oil, avocado oil is also rich in omega-6 and omega-3 fatty acids, making it slightly anti-inflammatory and helpful for balancing the tendency to consume too many omega-6 fatty acids, which may contribute to the increase in inflammatory disease. Avocado oil also has a zero impact on glycemic load.

There are claims that avocado oil fights heart disease, protects against diabetes, macular degeneration, prostate and other cancers. There are even claims that it reduces wrinkles. (It has been a beauty product and medicinal additive for many years.) The cold-pressed unrefined oil contains the highest level of monounsaturated fats and omega-3 fatty acids which lower blood cholesterol. It also contains the highest levels of alpha- and beta-caroten which protect against heart disease, twice the lutein of olive oil which protects against macular degeneration, and high levels of several essential vitamins and minerals including the powerful antioxidant, vitamin E.

Flaxseed Oil

The flaxseed plant, also called Linum usitatissimum, has its origin in Europe where it was a source of fibre. Gradually it came to be used as a healing herb and was often used in the place of what is now a multi-vitamin supplement. It is rich in omega-3 fatty acids (EFAs) and is touted to be useful in treating cardiac ailments and even lupus. The EFAs are the key components present in flaxseed oil because similar acids are required to protect cell membranes. The omega-3 acids are good for the heart and the omega-6 are similar to those found in vegetable oils.

Heart-healthy and loaded with cancer-fighting antioxidants, flax and flaxseed oil promise to follow soy to the supermarket shelves as the next powerhouse food. The main reason is that flaxseed is a super source of lignans, fibre and omega-3 fats. The concentration of lignans in flaxseed is more than 100 times greater than that found in any other lignan-containing foods such as grains, fruits and vegetables.

The health benefits of flaxseed oil are extensive. It controls high blood pressure, helps lower cholesterol and guards against heart disease. The benefits also extend to combating inflammation due to gout and inflammation in the joints and kidneys. The omega-3 acids present in flaxseed oil help to absorb the iodine and this is very useful in treating conditions where iodine is present in small amounts. It is also useful in controlling constipation. The dietary fibre content in the oil is considerable and helps ease bowel movements.

Flaxseed oil also helps alleviate skin problems. The EFAs target the sites of the inflammation and bring about an overall soothing. Acne, psoriasis, sunburn and rosaccea have all been known to respond favourably to flaxseed oil. The omega-3 acids ensure healthy hair and nails, and they also help to revitalize skin and prevent nails from cracking and breaking.

Flaxseed oil helps to reduce severity of nerve damage and also aids in triggering nerve impulses. It helps to combat the effects of aging and the lignans present in the oil guard against cancer. Another important area where it is of great help is the brain. The omega-3 fatty acids help retain emotional health, thereby helping to tackle depression and possibly Alzheimer's disease. Used externally, it can soften dry skin.

The oil has a low smoke point and is used in salads. It is also ingested in capsule form for various other disorders. Flaxseeds themselves can be crushed and used in beverages (such as juices and smoothies), bread and other baked products. The oil should be kept away from heat and light.

Oils

Grape Seed Oil

Grape seed oil is made from pomace, the waste left in the grape press during the winemaking process after the pressing cycle. The oil obtained from a further dehydration and pressing process is rich in nutrients, especially antioxidants and fatty acids like linoleic acid.

The nutritional components in grape seed oil provide a variety of health benefits, one of the most important being their ability to slow down and reserve free radical damage and reduce the risk of disease, especially heart disease. It also slows skin aging. Grape seed oil is a powerful antioxidant, fifty times more potent than vitamin E and twenty times more effective than vitamin C in destroying free radicals, harmful molecules that roam the body and damage cells.

Certain components in grape seed oil can help protect the body from sun damage, improve vision, flexibility in the joints, arteries and body tissue, improve blood circulation and reduce allergic and asthmatic symptoms by inhibiting the formation of histamines. Many studies have been carried out to determine the benefits of using grape seed oil and, today, it is used in controlling various health problems like heart disease and cancer and for regulating blood sugar levels. Grape seed oil is rich in vitamins E and C, flavonoids and beta-carotene.

Grape seed oil presumably lowers cholesterol, especially LDL ('bad') cholesterol. On the other hand, it has been found to increase HDL ('good') cholesterol, which reduces risks of coronary diseases. Some studies have shown that grape seed extract may be helpful in checking the growth of cancerous cells in the stomach, colon, prostate and lung. Certain compounds found in grape seed oil are believed to improve vision, flexibility of joints and blood circulation.

Grape seed oil is usually colourless with a high smoke point and is widely used in cooking. It can be used in baking, frying, salad dressings, marinades and sauces.

Olive Oil

Olive oil contains monounsaturated fat, a healthier type of fat that can lower your risk of heart disease by reducing the total and LDL ('bad') cholesterol levels in your blood, making it a healthier choice.

In contrast, saturated and trans fats such as butter, animal fats, tropical oils and partially hydrogenated oils, increase your risk of heart disease by increasing your total and bad cholesterol levels. All types of oils contain monounsaturated fat, but extra virgin or virgin olive oils are the least processed forms, so they are the most heart healthy. Olive oil is rich in antioxidants like chlorophyll, carotenoids and vitamin E. Scientists have identified a compound in olive oil called oleuropein, which prevents the LDL cholesterol from oxidizing. It is the oxidized cholesterol that sticks to the wall of the arteries and forms plaque. Replacing other fats in your diet with olive oil can significantly lower blood pressure and reduce the risk of heart attack.

A study published in the January 2005 issue of *Annals of Oncology* has identified oleic acid, a monounsaturated fatty acid found in olive oil, as having the ability to reduce the effect of an oncogene (a gene that will turn a host cell into a cancer cell). This particular oncogene is associated with the rapid growth of breast cancer tumours. The conclusion of the researchers was that oleic acid when combined with drug therapy encouraged the self-destruction of aggressive, treatment-resistant cancer cells thereby destroying the cancer. Olive oil has been positively indicated in studies of prostate and endometrial cancers as well. Unlike other fats, which are associated with the higher risk of colon cancer, olive oil helps protect the cells of the colon from carcinogens. A study published in the November 2003 issue of *Food Chemistry Toxicology* suggests that the antioxidants in olive oil reduce the amounts of carcinogens formed when meat is cooked.

Diabetics or those at risk of diabetes are advised to combine a low-fat, high-carbohydrate diet with olive oil. Studies show this combination is superior at controlling blood sugar levels compared to a diet that consists entirely of low-fat meals. Adding olive oil is also linked to lower triglyceride levels which put diabetics at risk of heart disease. The body uses the healthy fats in olive oil to produce natural anti-inflammatory agents which can help reduce the severity of both arthritis and asthma. Un-inflamed cell membranes are more fluid and better able to move healthy nutrients into the cells and move waste products out. A lower incidence of osteoporosis and dementia is found in areas where people consume large quantities of olive oil.

Do not place your bottle of olive oil on the windowsill. Light and heat are oil's

Oils

number one enemy. Keep your olive oil in a cool dark place, tightly sealed. Oxygen promotes rancidity and, when exposed to air, light or high temparatures, olive oil goes rancid. Olive oil has a higher smoke point than virgin and extra virgin olive oils, which makes it ideal for cooking. Virgin and extra virgin olive oils are best used for salads, dressing and dips.

Palm Oil

Palm oil has long been perceived as an unhealthy tropical oil, but it is actually a beneficial fat source when in its natural form. Palm oil comes from the pulp of the fruit of the Elaeis guineensis tree, also called the African palm oil tree. It has a red-orange colour and is popular in the preparation of dishes native to the Caribbean and West African countries.

Though palm oil is known for its high saturated fat content that is implicated in increasing the chances of heart disease, it also has nutritional benefits. Palm oil is a rich source of antioxidants. It is the richest vegetable source of tocotrienols, which are a potent source of Vitamin E. Vitamin E strengthens the immune system, protects skin cells from toxins and UV radiation, and helps protect against diseases such as cancer and blood disorders.

From its reddish-orange colour, palm oil is also a good source of beta-carotene, a nutrient found in sweet potatoes, carrots and other orange fruits. Beta-carotene is a very important form of vitamin A that by acting as an antioxidant helps protect our body against diseases like Alzheimer's, cataracts, arthritis and cancers. Palm oil also contains high-density lipoprotein (HDL), the good type of fat that helps protect against cholesterol. The key is to use palm oil in moderation.

Sesame Seed Oil

Derived from the sesame seed, sesame oil is perhaps best known as a common ingredient in Asian and East Indian cooking. Also known as gingelly, sesame oil has also been used for thousands of years as a popular alternative medical treatment in Ayurvedic and Oriental medicines. The oil is obtained from both raw seeds (cold pressed) and toasted seeds, and is valued for its long shelf life and high heat tolerance.

Historically, sesame oil has been used as an anti-inflammatory, antiseptic and pain-reliever in skin conditions, gum disease and a variety of other illnesses. Modern science now knows that sesame oil is a powerful antioxidant, high in polyunsaturated fats and an excellent source of vitamin E and minerals. Sesame oil, in fact, has the fourth highest concentration of polyunsaturated fats of any oil. Polyunsaturated fats are thought to be important in the prevention of illnesses such as diabetes, heart disease, high blood pressure, arthritis and autoimmune disorders. Because sesame oil is a natural, readily attainable source of these important polyunsaturated fats as well as because of its vitamin and antioxidant properties, it has begun to gain the interest of traditional western medicine. It has been the subject of multiple clinical studies and continues to be examined as a potential treatment for cancer, menopause, gum disease, high blood pressure and heart disease.

Sesame oil is known for its healing power. When used as a massage oil, it protects the skin from problems such as eczema, psoriasis and blemishes. It is an excellent emollient and is beneficial in alleviating tension and stress. It has been observed that people suffering from hypertension are usually prone to anxiety, poor circulation, nerve and bone disorders. Thus, application of the oil protects the body from various disorders associated with the nervous system. It also helps with insomnia and mental fatigue.

Oils

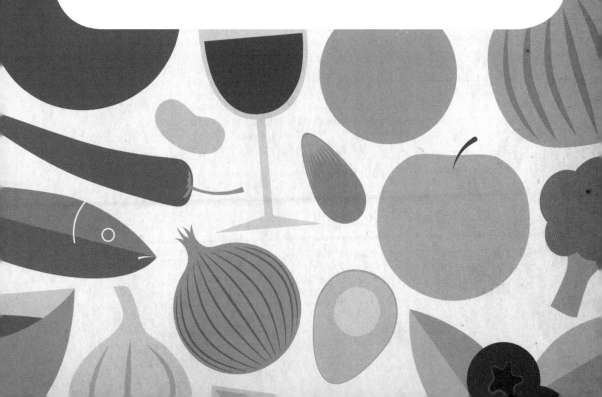

Chapter 3

Spices

There are a lot of spices on the market that have medicinal benefits in their own right. Many have been around since ancient times and have been used both for medicinal and culinary purposes. It is worth noting though that the more spices are used on a daily basis, the more beneficial their effects. Also, they work better in combination as certain spices enhance the nutritional benefits of others, for example a compound in black pepper enhances the effects of other spices such as turmeric.

Aniseed

Aniseed, or Illicium verum, is a native plant of Asia, commonly used in traditional societies to spice food, reduce intestinal gas, aid in digestion and act as a powerful diuretic medicinal herb. These aromatic seeds are used in confectionary and as flavouring for alcoholic beverages. They have a rich, pervasively spicy-sweet odour resembling liquorice.

Aniseed is potently therapeutic. Warming and enlivening the body, it can invigorate the mind and stimulate circulation. Its powerful action on the digestive system stems nausea and vomiting, and eases indigestion and flatulence. Its expectorant properties are also useful in treating respiratory infections. Aniseed is also known to promote vitality and vigour in the human system, and is a common ingredient in the French liqueur Pernod.

Basil

Basil is used extensively as a condiment in both Eastern and Western cuisines. The herb is used traditionally as a digestive aid and an antiseptic. A number of basil's phytochemicals have been well researched in other spices and are known to have important medicinal properties.

According to scientific studies, basil contains several potent anti-microbial chemicals. Ursolic acid and apigenin demonstrate strong activity against the herpes viruses, and apigenin is also effective against hepatitis viruses. Linalool helps fight adenoviruses that are responsible for the common cold and other respiratory infections like croup. The antioxidant, eugenol, inhibits platelet aggregation. The flavonoids in basil protect cell structures as well as chromosomes from radiation and oxygen-based damage. Basil has anti-inflammatory effects, making it an ideal food for those people suffering from arthritis. Basil oil contains eugenol, which blocks the activity of an enzyme in the body called cyclooxygenase that normally causes swelling.

Basil is a rich source of beta-carotene which helps protect epithelial cells (the lining of numerous body structures including the blood vessels) from free radical damage. It is also a good source of magnesium, a mineral that makes the muscles and blood vessels relax, thereby improving blood flow and lessening the risk of irregular heart rhythm. Basil is a very good source of iron, calcium, potassium and vitamins C and K, and dietary fibres.

Bay Leaves

Although the bay leaf was not introduced to England until the sixteenth century, it has been around since ancient Greek and Roman times. It was held in such high esteem that victors of battle, sport and study were crowned with garlands of bay leaves (also known as laurel), as a symbol of their success.

Bay leaves are a good source of vitamins A and C, and also contain significant amounts of iron and manganese in particular, as well as smaller amounts of calcium, potassium and magnesium. In ancient times, bay leaves were used medicinally for a number of ailments such as liver, kidney and stomach problems, and were also thought to heal wasp and bee stings.

Bay leaf contains caffeic acid, quercetin, eugenol and catechins, all of which have chemo-protective properties against several different types of cancer. As an important component of Mediterranean seasonings, bay leaves contain valuable compounds that contribute to the cardiovascular health benefits associated with the Mediterranean diet.

Black Peppercorns

Black pepper is derived from the fruit of a climbing vine native to Southern India and Sri Lanka. Used almost universally, it is one of the most common condiments worldwide. One of black pepper's most important attributes is its ability to improve digestion. It actually stimulates taste buds to notify the stomach to increase its secretion of hydrochloric acid thereby improving the digestion of food once it reaches your stomach – so load up on black pepper! Personally, I can't cook anything without it.

The antioxidant property of black pepper prevents and curtails oxidative stress. Moreover, several of these compounds work indirectly by enhancing the action of other antioxidants. It also reduces the damage caused by a diet full of saturated fats, which is found to be the main cause of oxidative stress. Black pepper also prevents bacterial growth in the intestinal tract.

Black pepper is effective against cancer. It counteracts the development of cancer directly by enhancing the cancer-fighting abilities of other spices. Its principle phytochemical, piperine, enhances the effects (bioavailability) of other compounds and spices such as curcumin in turmeric to inhibit some of the pro-inflammatory cytokines that are produced by tumour cells, hence reducing the chances of tumour progression.

Cardamom

Cardamom is one of the most important spices in many Eastern cuisines and is used in some Middle Eastern countries for flavouring coffee. It is also used as a breath freshener. As one of the most expensive of the spices, cardamom is exceeded in price only by saffron and vanilla.

Studies have shown that cardamom possess the ability to kill harmful H. pylori bacteria associated with ulcers. It also has a calming effect on the rest of the digestive tract and has been used to treat indigestion and gastritis (inflammation of the lining of the stomach).

Cardamom is best purchased and stored in whole pod form because once the seeds are exposed or ground, they quickly lose their flavour. It can be added to rice pudding and other milk-based dishes.

Chilli

Chilli peppers contain a substance called capsaicin, which gives them their characteristic pungence and produces mild to intense spice when eaten. Capsaicin is a potent inhibitor of substance P, a neuropeptide associated with inflammatory process. The hotter the chilli pepper, the more capsaicin it contains. The hottest varieties include habanero and Scotch bonnet peppers. Jalapenos come next in their heat and capsaicin content, followed by the milder varieties, including Spanish pimentos, Anaheim and Hungarian cherry peppers.

Red chilli peppers, such as cayenne, have been shown to reduce blood cholesterol, triglyceride levels and platelet aggregation, while increasing the body's ability to dissolve fibrin, a substance integral to the formation of blood clots. Cultures where hot pepper is used liberally have a much lower rate of heart attack, stroke and pulmonary embolism.

Capsaicin not only reduces pain, but its peppery heat also stimulates secretions that help clear mucus from your stuffed-up nose or congested lungs. The chilli pepper's bright red colour signals its high content of beta-carotene or pro-vitamin A. Just two teaspoons of red chilli peppers provide about six percent of the recommended daily value for vitamin C coupled with more than ten percent of the daily value for vitamin A. Often called the anti-infection vitamin, vitamin A is essential for healthy mucous membranes which line the nasal passages, lungs, intestinal tract and urinary tract, and serves as the body's first defence against invading germs.

The capsaicin in red chilli peppers stops the spread of prostate cancer cells through a variety of mechanisms, indicated in a study published in a 2006 issue of *Cancer Research*. Capsaicin triggers suicide in both primary types of prostate cancer cell line, those whose growth is stimulated by male hormones and those not affected by them.

Chives

Chives are the onion family's smallest species. They are called chives as they always grow in clumps. They are native to North America, Europe and Asia. Chives are mainly used for culinary purposes especially in soups and dishes using potatoes and fish.

The use of chives as a medicine is similar to that of garlic, only a little weaker. Chives help improve blood circulation and lower blood pressure. They are also a good source of vitamins A and C, calcium, potassium and folic acid. The best-known benefit of chives is that they reduce the growth of tumours and cancer. They are helpful in stomach and esophageal cancer as well as prostate cancer, although you would need to consume a lot to get the medicinal benefits.

Cinnamon

Cinnamon is a tree that grows in India, Sri Lanka, Indonesia, Brazil, Vietnam and Egypt. It is one of the oldest spices, known since ancient times. To prepare it, the bark of the cinnamon tree is dried and rolled into cinnamon sticks, also called quills, which is known as 'real' cinnamon (cinnamon zeylanicum). Cinnamon can also be dried and ground into powder form.

In traditional Chinese medicine, a different type of cinnamon (known as cinnamon cassia) is used for colds, flatulence, nausea, diarrhoea and painful menstrual periods. It is also believed to improve energy, vitality and circulation, and to be particularly useful for people, like me, who tend to feel hot in their upper body but have cold feet. I often use cinnamon sticks in my tea during winter and it does help with the cold feet syndrome.

Cinnamon is an excellent source of manganese, dietary fibre, iron and calcium. Antioxidants found in cinnamon include epicatechin, camphene, eugenol, phenol, salicylic acid and tannins. A study of the antioxidant properties of spices determined that adding flavouring substances such as cinnamon in the preparation of tea (including black tea and green tea) enhanced its total antioxidant activities – a welcome additional benefit.

Cinnamon is a powerful inducer of insulin sensitivity making it an effective treatment for both type 2 diabetes and metabolic syndrome. In his book, *Medicinal Seasonings*, author Dr Keith Scott indicates that recent landmark clinical trials have shown that the daily addition of as little as one gram of cinnamon to the diet leads to a reduction of blood glucose levels of between 18 and 29 percent in type 2 diabetics. In a study published by researchers at the U.S. Department of Agriculture in Maryland, cinnamon reduced the proliferation of leukaemia and lymphoma cancer cells. It has an anti-clotting effect on the blood. The results from a study at the Nutrient Requirements and Functions Laboratory suggest the potential of polyphenols from cinnamon in inhibiting tumour cell proliferation.

Coriander

Coriander is a powerful herb with many health benefits. Commonly known as cilantro, this leafy herb is used in most cuisines. Originating in the Mediterranean region, it thrives in black soil and arid regions.

Coriander leaves contain protein, fat, minerals, fibre, carbohydrates and water. The minerals and vitamins include vitamin C, calcium, phosphorus, iron, carotene, thiamine, riboflavin, niacin, sodium, potassium and oxalic acid. The leaves act as stimulants; they strengthen the stomach and promote digestion, increase secretion and discharge of urine and reduce fever. The juice of coriander is beneficial in producing vitamins A, B1 and B2, and iron. Coriander seeds are known to alleviate excessive menstrual flow. Dried coriander is excellent in treating conjunctivitis. It relieves burning and reduces pain and swelling.

Coriander's anti-tumorigenic properties have been demonstrated in relation to colon cancer. It works by protecting against the damaging effects of lipid oxidation associated with this malignancy. It is highly probable that coriander also contributes to the low incidences of several other types of cancer seen in the populations of Eastern nations that consume it in large quantities.

Coriander lowers cholesterol and triglyceride levels, helping to reduce the risk of atherosclerosis and thereby heart attack and stroke. It does this through two mechanisms: by inhibiting the uptake of these lipids in the intestines, and by enhancing their breakdown and excretion.

Cumin

Native to the Eastern Mediterranean region, this spice has been used by humans since ancient times. In ancient Egypt, cumin was added to food as a condiment and used in the mummification of the dead. The Romans and ancient Greeks likewise used cumin in cooking and also for cosmetic purposes, and it is mentioned in the Bible as a form of payment. Today, cumin is an important component of a variety of cuisines, including Middle Eastern, Indian, North African and South American.

Cumin has been used traditionally as an analgesic and also to treat indigestion. The seeds themselves are rich in iron and are thought to help stimulate the secretion of enzymes from the pancreas, which can help absorb nutrients into the system. It has also been shown to boost the power of the liver's ability to detoxify the body. Recent studies have revealed that cumin seeds might also have anti-carcinogenic properties. In laboratory tests, this powerful little seed was shown to reduce the risk of stomach and liver tumours in animals.

The health benefits of cumin for digestive disorders have been well-known throughout history. It can help with flatulence, indigestion, diarrhoea, nausea, morning sickness and atonic dyspepsia. Cumin is also said to help relieve the symptoms of the common cold due to its antiseptic properties.

Curry Leaves

The curry leaf comes from a shrub native to India and is an important ingredient in spicy Eastern dishes. Ironically, it is not always added to the curry powders in the west, which generally consist of a combination of other spices such as cumin, coriander, black pepper, ginger and fenugreek.

The curry leaf contains the antiviral compounds linalool and limonene, which have also demonstrated protective effects against some cancers. Curry leaves in general can stimulate salivary secretions, which in turn initiate the secretion of digestive juices. In South India, curry leaves are used to control blood sugar in non-insulin dependent diabetics.

The fruit from the curry tree are purplish berries. The juice from these berries mixed with lime juice forms an acidic and effective solution for external relief from insect bites and stings.

Fennel Seeds

Fennel seeds have a similar flavour to aniseed or liquorice and are quite strong. They are used in many European dishes to flavour fish, bread and confectionaries. The more subtly-flavoured stalks are widely used as a vegetable and in salads. In ancient Greece, fennel was known as 'marathon', because it grew at the famous battle site, and it was used as a symbol of victory.

Fennel contains a variety of important vitamins, nutrients and antioxidants, including limonene which has anti-cancer properties. It is an excellent source of folate, fibre and potassium. These nutrients are essential for good colon and cardiovascular health. The health benefits of fennel also include keeping cholesterol and blood pressure levels down. Fennel can help reduce the discomfort associated with menstruation by regulating the hormonal activity. Nursing mothers, with the supervision of their doctors, can use fennel to help increase milk production.

The high amounts of phytonutrients and vitamin C can help neutralize free radicals in the body, helping to prevent cancer and other degenerative health conditions.

Fenugreek

Fenugreek seeds are the most valuable part of the plant and have long been used as a nourishing dietary spice in the Middle East, India and the Far East. It is also an important constituent of curries. In traditional medicine, fenugreek has been used to treat a number of conditions including diabetes and sore throats, and in poultices used to treat sores and abscesses. Recent investigations into the medicinal properties of this spice suggest it is important not only as a prevention for chronic diseases such as diabetes, but also for enhancing normal physiological processes, especially with respect to athletic performance.

Fenugreek is one of the richest sources of selenium, which is among the most important antioxidant micronutrients. When consumed regularly, selenium appears to have a protective effect against a range of cancers, including those of the colon, lung and prostate.

Fenugreek is rich in vitamins A and D, and also contains smaller amounts of vitamins B1, B2 and B3. It contains oil that is similar to cod liver oil and is high in protein. It also contains the minerals choline and iron and some lecithin. Fenugreek works on softening hardened mucous and helps to cleanse toxic waste through the lymphatic system. It helps clear mucous from the lungs and bowels.

Fenugreek helps to alleviate type 2 diabetes. According to one study, it may help people with type 1 diabetes as well. A study carried out by Indian researchers revealed that fenugreek added to a type 1 diabetic's diet helps drop urinary sugar levels by 54 percent. Because of the presence of the natural fibre galactomannan, fenugreek slows down the rate at which sugar is absorbed into the blood. The amino acid (4-hydroxyisoleucine) in fenugreek induces the production of insulin. Therefore, 15 to 20 grams of fenugreek daily is recommended for controlling blood sugar.

Fenugreek possesses anti-carcinogenic properties. The steroid, diosgenin, in fenugreek is colon cancer protective. Fenugreek is also used to treat wounds, inflammation and gastrointestinal ailments. It helps in antioxidation, so prevents and repairs damage caused by free radicals. According to Ayurvedic and Chinese medicines, fenugreek can be used for inducing labour and aiding digestion. It is also good for improving metabolism and health, and soothes irritated skin conditions when applied externally.

Garam Masala

Garam masala is actually a mixture of different spices that are added to many Indian dishes. Typically, garam masala includes cumin, coriander, cardamom, black pepper and cinnamon, but may also include bay leaves.

The combination of spices offers many beneficial properties. Cinnamon is anti-microbial and anti-inflammatory and it may help boost brain function and control blood sugar in people with diabetes. Cumin is an excellent source of iron. It aids digestion and has cancer-fighting properties. Coriander is sometimes referred to as an anti-diabetic plant because it helps control blood sugar. It also has anti-inflammatory properties and it helps lower cholesterol (see above for more information on the spices used in making garam masala).

Garlic

Garlic, the bulb of a plant native to the Himalayas and Siberia, is among the world's most important spices both from a culinary and medicinal perspective. Used across the globe as a pungent food flavouring, in many societies garlic is used as an important medicinal spice with an array of traditional uses. These include its use as an antiseptic, anti-asthmatic, anti-rheumatic and as a treatment for coughs and colds.

In his book *Medicinal Seasonings*, Dr Scott explains that the regular consumption of garlic has a protective effect against a number of different malignancies, including cancers of the colon, breast, bladder, liver, prostate, lung and leukaemia. He identifies that garlic also inhibits helicobacter pylori infection of the stomach, preventing ulceration caused by this bacterium and thereby reducing the risk of stomach cancer.

A large-scale epidemiological Iowa Women's Health study looked at the garlic consumption in 41,000 middle-aged women. Results showed that women who regularly consumed garlic had a 35 percent lower risk of developing colon cancer. Many of the health benefits of garlic that have been studied come from garlic's abundant antioxidant nutrients. Garlic contains enzymes, calcium, copper, iron, manganese, phosphorus, potassium and selenium. Vitamins in garlic include vitamins A, B1 (thiamine), B2 (riboflavin), B6 and C. Garlic also contains dozens of bioflavonoids, more than 80 sulphur-containing compounds.

Garlic has been shown to fight bacterial infections, boost the immune system, balance blood sugar levels, assist in fat metabolism and reduce high blood pressure. Studies have shown that the benefits of garlic extend to the prevention of cancer. Although scientists don't know why exactly garlic has the ability to prevent cancer, an examination of the amazing phytonutrient content of garlic gives us good reason to believe that garlic could be a potent anti-cancer food. Studies around the world have shown that people who ate more garlic had a significantly lower incidence of cancer. Typically, these people ate more garlic than most people would want to because of its strong aroma: five cloves or more a day. However, with the availability of odour-free garlic capsules today, there is no reason to avoid adding garlic to your healthy diet.

Ginger

Dishes made with ginger, onion and garlic combinations are popular in Northern Indian cuisine. Ginger is used for its warming properties, unique taste and aroma.

Ginger contains gingerol, a compound that is thought to relax blood vessels, stimulate blood flow and relieve pain. It is commonly used as a digestive aid and contains compounds that ease motion sickness and nausea, and inhibit vomiting. This makes it a helpful spice for morning sickness or for people suffering from the side effects of chemotherapy. Ginger is high in antioxidants and also has anti-inflammatory properties, which means it may be useful in fighting heart disease, cancer, Alzheimer's disease and arthritis.

Ginger may be a powerful weapon in the treatment of ovarian cancer. A study conducted at the University of Michigan Comprehensive Cancer Center found that ginger powder induced cell death in all ovarian cancer cells to which it was applied. Another study at the University of Minnesota found that ginger may slow the growth of colorectal cancer cells. A component of ginger suppresses metastasis (i.e. stops the spread) in any type of cancer cell including leukaemia, skin, kidney, lung and pancreatic cancer cells – one of the most exciting and powerful health benefits of ginger.

Ginger can also be used in treating the common cold. By adding a few slices to hot water with lemon and honey, it helps to ease congestion and cleanses the body.

Mint

Mints are widely used as digestive aids in the form of teas and are important for their culinary uses. Certain mints, especially peppermint, have some of the most potent antioxidant properties of all spices. These include rosmarinic acid, which inhibits plaque formation in the arteries. Mints also contain limonene, which provides protection against some cancers. The strong and refreshing aroma of mint is an excellent and quick remedy for nausea. Many people keep mentha oil or mint flavoured products with them to avoid nausea, particularly when they are travelling. Mint balms or mint oil, when rubbed on the forehead or nose, give quick headache relief.

While mint oil is a good antiseptic, mint juice is an excellent skin cleanser. It soothes skin, cures infections, itching, etc., and is also good for acne. Its antipruritic properties can be used for treating insect bites such as those from mosquitoes, honey bees, hornets and wasps. Being a germicidal and breath freshener, it takes care of oral health by inhibiting harmful bacterial growth inside your mouth.

Current research shows that enzymes present in mint may help cure cancer because of their anti-cancer properties. The phytonutrient, perillyl alcohol, is believed to prevent colon, skin and lung cancer. Another peculiar property, which is very much contrary to mint's cooling and soothing effects, is that it induces sweating if consumed during fever, thereby curing it. Mint juice can be applied to burns to heal and soothe them. It is also beneficial in rheumatism and is said to improve brain activity, although there is, at present, insufficient proof.

Mustard Seeds

Mustard seed is a powerful anti-microbial agent which can kill E. coli bacteria, listeria and other foodborne pathogens.

Mustard seeds are a very good source of selenium, a nutrient which has been shown to help reduce the severity of asthma, decrease some of the symptoms of rheumatoid arthritis and help prevent cancer. They also qualify as a good source of magnesium. Like selenium, magnesium has been shown to help reduce the severity of asthma, lower high blood pressure, restore normal sleep patterns in women having difficulty with the symptoms of menopause, reduce the frequency of migraines, and to prevent heart attacks in patients suffering from atherosclerosis or diabetic heart disease.

Mustard seeds are also a very good source of omega-3 fatty acids, iron, calcium, zinc, manganese, magnesium, protein, niacin and dietary fibre. They contain high amounts of phytonutrients called glucosinolates. The seeds also contain myrosinase enzymes that can break the glucosinolates apart into other phytonutrients called isothiocyanates. The isothiocyanates in mustard seeds have been repeatedly studied for their anti-cancer effects. In animal studies and particularly in studies involving the gastrointestinal tract and colorectal cancer, intake of isothiocyanates has been shown to inhibit the growth of existing cancer cells and protect against the formation of such cells.

Mustard seeds may be added to hot ghee (clarified butter used in Indian cuisine) to lend a nutty flavour to many dishes. They are also used as flavouring for vegetables and lentils.

Nutmeg

Nutmeg is used to flavour confectionary as well as many savoury and sweet dishes. It also has some traditional medicinal uses, including as a treatment for diarrhoea. In high doses, it has narcotic effects.

Nutmeg provides several important antioxidants, including eugenol which inhibits platelet aggregation and oleanolic acid which can lower blood lipids. It also contains limonene which, as mentioned previously, has preventive properties against some cancers, and linalool which has anti-cancer and antiviral effects.

Nutmeg is known to have anti-inflammatory properties and can be used to treat joint and muscle pain. The oil works particularly well for this when it is massaged into the affected area. It is an integral herb in Chinese medicine in which it is used for stomach pain and inflammation as well as reducing joint swelling.

Paprika

Paprika is unusually high in vitamin C. Hungary's Nobel Prize-winning Professor Szent-Györgyi first discovered the vitamin in paprika chilli peppers. The bell (capsicum) peppers used for paprika contain six to nine times as much vitamin C as tomatoes by weight. High heat degrades the vitamin content of peppers, meaning that commercially dried peppers are not as nutritious as those dried naturally in the sun.

As an anti-bacterial agent and stimulant, paprika can help normalize blood pressure, improve circulation and increase the production of saliva and stomach acids to aid digestion.

Saffron

Known as a golden and expensive spice, saffron is indeed a very special and precious spice with numerous health benefits. It is particularly used in cooking to add an aroma and spice to food as it has the quality of turning any dish into an exotic one.

Saffron has numerous health benefits. It has long been used for improving digestion and appetite, and the treatment of kidney, bladder and liver disorders as it helps improve circulation to the digestive organs. Also, it coats the membranes of the stomach and colon thereby helping to soothe gastrointestinal colic and acidity. Saffron is found to be extremely beneficial for providing relief from gas and acid related problems.

It helps in treating various disorders such as asthma, atherosclerosis, painful menstrual periods and even depression, amongst others. The spice is considered as a blood purifier and anti-inflammatory. It helps in relieving inflammation of arthritis along with providing relief from joint pains. It is also said to be a mild sedative which can be used for insomnia and even to treat depression.

Cooking with saffron is popular in the Middle East, Spain and Italy. It has a wonderful aroma and also adds colour to the food. Saffron contains carotenoids, which are known to inhibit skin tumours and improve arthritis in various independent studies. The numerous active constituents in saffron are also known to bring about a positive effect on people with neurodegenerative disorders and memory problems. Massaging the gums with saffron helps in reducing soreness and inflammation of the mouth and tongue.

Saffron is usually used in its dried form and is expensive as a spice and as a herbal supplement. When choosing saffron as a herbal supplement, opt for whole saffron threads as they tend to have more medicinal properties than the powder.

Saffron may have anti-cancer effects and it also helps in lowering LDL ('bad') cholesterol. Additionally, saffron acts as an antispasmodic and is used in cough suppressants. It also aids in the treatment of whooping cough, acidity, headaches, acne and urinary disorders among others. Research has found anti-cancerous properties in saffron. This is primarily due to antioxidants present in it which provide protection against various kinds of cancers such as leukaemia and ovarian carcinoma, and which also provide protection against coronary heart disease, diabetes and hepatitis.

Sesame Seeds

Sesame seeds are a good source of manganese and copper. They are also a good source of calcium, magnesium, iron, phosphorus, vitamin B1, zinc and dietary fibre. In addition to these important nutrients, sesame seeds contain two unique substances: sesamin and sesamolin. Both these substances belong to a group of phyto-oestrogens called lignans, and have been shown to have a cholesterol-lowering effect in humans, and to prevent high blood pressure and increase vitamin E supplies in animals. Sesamin has also been found to protect the liver from oxidative damage.

Tahini

Tahini may be made from hulled or un-hulled sesame seeds. The tahini made with un-hulled sesame seeds is richer in vitamins and minerals but is darker and has a stronger flavour, so it may not suit some recipes. Because the sesame seeds are ground into a paste, tahini is easy to digest, and within half an hour of its consumption it provides the body with a balanced supply of energy, vitamins and minerals.

Tahini, being rich in vitamins A, E and B, biotin and choline is a nutritional powerhouse. It is also 20 percent complete protein making it a richer protein source than milk, soy beans, sunflower seeds and most nuts. Tahini has one of the highest sources of methionine, an essential amino acid, and also contains lecithin, which reduces the levels of fat in the blood and also protects against environmental toxins such as nicotine. Tahini is also high in minerals such as magnesium, potassium, iron and phosphorus, and is an excellent source of calcium. In fact, tahini is claimed to be the best source of calcium there is and, unlike dairy products that also supply calcium, it is not mucous forming.

Turmeric

Turmeric comes from the root of the Curcuma longa plant and has a tough brown skin and a deep orange flesh. Turmeric has long been used as a powerful anti-inflammatory in both the Chinese and Indian systems of medicine to treat a wide variety of conditions including flatulence, jaundice, menstrual difficulties, bloody urine, haemorrhage, toothache, bruises, chest pain and colic.

Curcumin's antioxidant actions, the main phytonutrient in turmeric, enable it to protect the colon cells from free radicals that can damage cellular DNA, a significant benefit particularly as cell turnover is quite rapid in the colon, occurring approximately every three days. Because of their frequent replication, mutations in the DNA of colon cells can result in the formation of cancerous cells, so curcumin helps prevent them from spreading through the body and causing more harm. A primary way in which curcumin does this is by enhancing liver function. Additionally, other suggested mechanisms by which it may protect against cancer development include inhibiting the synthesis of a protein thought to be instrumental in tumour formation and preventing the development of additional blood supply necessary for cancer cell growth. Turmeric or curcumin is one of the most-researched spices regarding cancer. But curcumin is not well-utilized by the body – it needs compounds like piperine (from black pepper) to protect it from being degraded by the body's digestive enzymes.

Spices

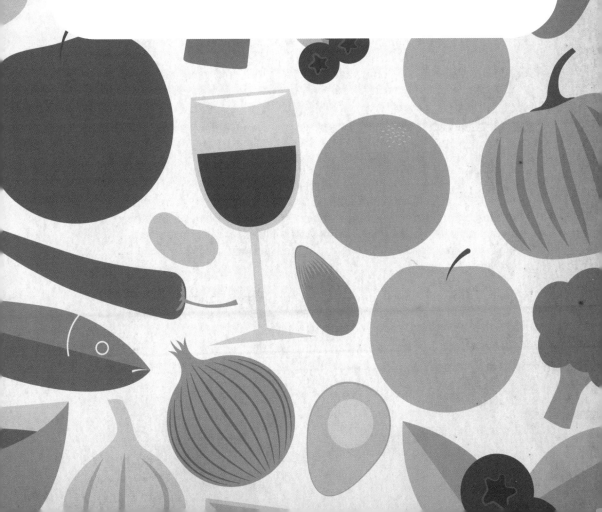

Chapter 4

Healthy Sweeteners

There are a lot of sweeteners out there
on the market, some good, others not so good.
I have chosen the two listed because of their
health benefits and low glycemic index (GI).

Agave Nectar

Agave nectar is a natural sweetener similar to honey and can be used to sweeten food and drink. This sweet syrup is an ideal alternative to sugar and is a healthier choice as it has a low glycemic index (GI) of 27 as opposed to honey's GI of 83.

The agave plant has long been cultivated in the hilly, semi-arid soils of Mexico. Its fleshy leaves cover the pineapple-shaped heart of the plant, which contains a sweet sticky juice. Ancient Mexicans considered the agave to be sacred. They believed the liquid from the plant purified body and soul.

According to Dr Sahelian, author of several books including *The Stevia Cookbook*, agave contains saponins and fructans, which have anti-inflammatory and immune system-boosting properties, including antimicrobial capability.

Agave can now be found in many supermarkets. I use agave nectar syrup from The Groovy Food Company, www.groovyfood.co.uk. You can get the syrup and other products from this company, from regular grocery and health food stores like Tesco, Waitrose and Holland & Barrett. More information on agave can be found at www.blueagavenectar.com.

Manuka Honey

Manuka honey is a premium medical-grade honey, exclusively found in New Zealand. It has been discovered that this unique type of honey has extraordinary healing properties that are capable of treating a wide spectrum of health conditions such as ulcers, acid reflux, acne, wounds, burns, eczema, MRSA Staph infections, etc. According to biochemist Peter Molan of the University of Waikato, manuka honey is rich in antibacterial properties. He and his colleagues have also suggested several benefits of manuka honey, including treatment of sore throats if taken orally.

Manuka honey can be found in some supermarkets and most health food shops.

Chapter 5

Acid to Placid

By Samantha Russo

Digestive disorders are on the increase and they are not alone: degenerative and chronic disorders are also on the incline. Disorders like coeliac disease, Crohn's disease, colitis, gastritis, fibromyalgia and chronic fatigue syndrome (CFS) are rapidly increasing in number, and some of them are fairly modern diseases that were not really heard of 100 years ago. All of these, if not treated, can lead to cancer.

A lot boils down to our diets – lacking in nutrients, with an over-reliance on processed and heavily-refined foods – environmental pollution and stress-filled days. All of these elements are taking their toll on our overworked systems.

This lifestyle can lead to an increase in the build-up of mucous plaque, which coats the colon, allowing bacteria to breed and stopping essential nutrients from being absorbed. To help avoid such problems and to re-energise your health with some gentleness, why not begin a journey from acid to placid?

To begin with you may experience some discomfort, but that's totally normal when your body is readjusting to love and tenderness. Here are the few basic principles of 'pain-free eating'.

Eat as much high water content produce (fresh fruit and vegetables) as possible

You know the saying, 'You are what you eat'. Well, my new saying is 'Eat what you are'. Our bodies are made up of predominantly water and the following indicates exactly how this is so:

- Saliva is 95 percent water
- Blood is 90 percent water
- Bone is 22 percent water
- Lean muscle tissue is 75 percent water
- Lymph is 94 percent water
- Lungs and brain are 80 percent water

As the body is largely made up of water, it is only obvious that it needs water to help keep it healthy and functioning properly. This is not just about drinking the minimum 8–10 cups of water each day, it's about eating foods that are naturally full of water such as fresh fruit and vegetables. They give your body the water it needs to help keep all your tissues hydrated and moist which is imperative in creating and maintaining your health. So, first, all the nutrients and vitamins found in fresh fruit and vegetables are transported to the intestines by the water in those fruit and vegetables, where they are absorbed and used by the body. Secondly, that same water that brought the nutrients in also carries the toxic wastes away from the body. As well as that, most fresh fruit and vegetables are alkaline foods, which help your body achieve and maintain an alkaline pH (7.35).

A few simple suggestions:

- Instead of potato with your lunch (chips, etc), have carrot sticks or cucumber and celery slices.
- If you are still hungry at the end of a meal, have seconds of tossed green salad instead of anything else.
- Make sure you serve a tray of raw veggies at all parties.
- If the children are hungry after school, give them fresh fruit instead of cookies, crisps or chips.
- Add chopped celery, cucumbers, onions and peppers to tuna or egg salad.
- Take veggie dippers (cut carrots, cucumbers, cherry tomatoes, broccoli, cauliflower, celery, radishes, peppers, courgettes) to work to nibble on instead of bending to the vending machine.

Correctly combine your food

Stop looking for that magic pill that will justify you eating chemical potions designed to taste unbelievably delicious. If you exist mainly on nutritionally-devoid, chemical-laden junk and expect to feel and look good or have more energy than a couch potato, think again. You need to stop complaining and stop taking pills for stomach problems, aches and pains and high cholesterol (among other things). All this can be eliminated (or immensely improved) by properly combining your meals.

If you suffer from a disease such as cancer, heart disease, arthritis or diabetes, listen here: your diet plays a major role in the development and severity of those diseases. Cancer cannot exist in a clean environment! It can only survive in a toxic environment. Waste that has not been eliminated from the body makes your body toxic. (Remember that fruit and vegetables help to eliminate waste.)

For example, uric acid is one of the most potent poisons in existence – and high protein foods (specifically animal products) are a major source of it. When uric acid settles in your joints, it leads to arthritis. Uric acid does not exist in fruit and vegetables. Basically, your body needs to be fed with high water-content foods. You absolutely cannot be healthy and free from diseases without them.

The concept of proper food combining has been around since 1911, believe it or not. But it's astounding how few people are aware of it or the importance of it. The idea was originated by Dr William Howard Hay, a New York physician who graduated from NYU Medical College in 1891 and who spent 16 years specializing in surgery. He then developed what is often a fatal kidney condition called Bright's disease, and after having no success with traditional medicine, he set out to find alternative methods to cure himself of the disease. He came up with the idea of food combining, which concerns itself with eating in such a way as to be in harmony with the physiological manner in which different foods are digested by the human body. That is, certain foods need an acid digestive enzyme, whereas other foods need an alkaline environment. So the two should not be mixed if fast, efficient digestion is to be achieved. Dr Hay cured his Bright's disease with this system of eating (now called the Hay Diet) and went on to become a famous author and lecturer.

The concept of food combining has since been adapted by many successful health practitioners, researchers and advisors. So basically, our bodies digest different foods in different ways. Fresh (non-starchy) vegetables, since they are largely made up of water, are a more 'neutral' type of food and pass through the stomach quickly with little or no digestive enzymes necessary. Starchy foods need an alkaline digestive enzyme, which starts in the mouth with the enzyme ptyalin and continues in the stomach and small intestine. Protein foods are digested by acid, specifically, hydrochloric acid and pepsin secreted by the stomach.

When an acid and an alkaline are mixed together in a lab beaker, they neutralize each other. The same concept applies in your stomach: when acid and alkaline digestive enzymes are mixed together in your stomach, they neutralize each other and, as a result, proper digestion is seriously damaged or completely stopped. With no working digestive enzymes to break it down, all that undigested food sits there in your stomach for six, seven, eight or even 14 hours and ferments, rots and putrefies until it's literally forced into the small intestine (by your next meal). That leads to gas, heartburn, cramps, bloating, flatulence, diarrhoea, and the list goes on. All this takes huge amounts of energy, so all you want to do is find the nearest place to curl up for a snooze!

Avoid processed foods and cut down on animal products

There are endless studies documenting the relationship between the consumption of animal products (including all meats, poultry, fish, milk, dairy products and animal fats) and the development of disease and obesity. High cholesterol is publicized as being one of the primary disease-causing factors. An interesting fact, however, is that cholesterol does not exist in plants. It is only found in the tissues of animals. Plus, plant foods are naturally high in fibre and low in fat, which are the most common characteristics suggested as necessary for a healthy diet. Animal products are high in fat and low in fibre – the exact opposite of what is considered 'healthy' by many authorities.

The most harmful and insulting to the human body are processed foods of any description. Basically, processed 'foods' are anything that comes in a jar, box, tin, can or bag with mile-long, hard to pronounce ingredients. Many have an indefinite shelf life in your cupboards, and they don't go off within a few days of you buying them the way 'real food' does.

Processed foods start off with 'real food' ingredients … but then those ingredients are completely destroyed and violated through one or more processes such as bleaching, fragmenting, heating, drying, freeze drying, evaporating and so on and so forth, until they in no way shape or form bear any resemblance to the 'real food' they started off as. Then various chemicals are added that serve a plethora of purposes – colouring, preservatives, artificial flavours, appearance enhancers, texture modifiers – plus some good old vitamins and nutrients are thrown in for good measure since the original ones in the food have been processed out.

Maintain an alkaline pH

Here is a brief explanation of what pH is and the importance of making sure yours is alkaline (7.35 is ideal). pH (potential of hydrogen) is the measure of hydrogen ions present in a solution. In non-biochemist terms, that means how acid or alkaline something is on a scale of 0–14, with 0 as extremely acid, 14 as extremely alkaline and 7 as neutral. Our blood naturally has a pH of 7.365, that is, slightly alkaline. And since blood is our life force nourishing all our organs and tissues, it is crucial to maintain its alkaline pH. Our pH is primarily the result of the food we eat. Other factors like stress and exercise can affect pH, but far and away the biggest factor affecting pH is our diet. The good news is that a perfect alkaline (about 7.35) is pretty easy to achieve and maintain. There are just three steps.

1. Check your pH regularly. You can purchase a saliva or urine test kit from most pharmacies and health shops. The saliva test is less accurate and urine is slightly more accurate. Alternatively, you can have a blood test carried out by a doctor, which is the most accurate but also the most expensive.

2. Drink loads of water – aim for at least 8–10 cups per day. Add a little lemon juice to make it more alkaline. Water is healthy and helps to flush away the toxins.

3. Eat a diet of at least 70 percent alkaline foods and properly combine all your meals. Fruit and vegetables such as cabbage, celery, parsley, spinach, tomatoes, summer squash, etc. are alkaline foods. A combination of vegetables and proteins gives abdominal comfort, e.g. fish with vegetables.

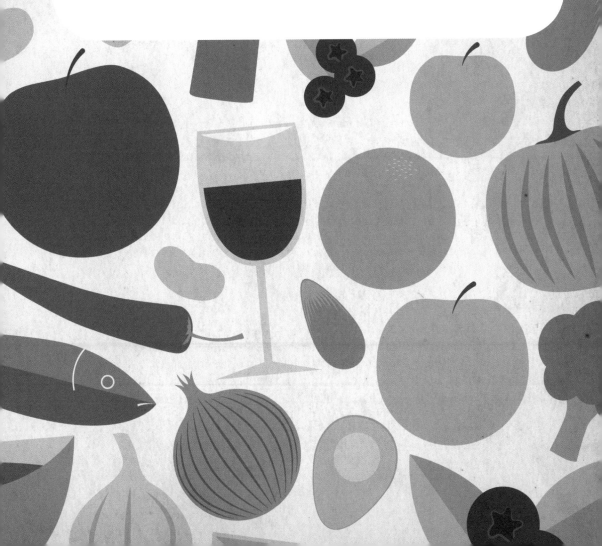

Chapter 6

Glossary

Here are definitions of some
commonly used words in this book.

Antioxidants

Antioxidants are molecules which can safely interact with free radicals to terminate the chain reaction before vital molecules are damaged. Although there are several enzyme systems within the body that scavenge free radicals, the principal micronutrient (vitamin) antioxidants are vitamins E and C and beta-carotene. Additionally, selenium, a trace mineral that is required for the proper function of one of the body's antioxidant enzyme systems, is sometimes included in this category. The body cannot manufacture these micronutrients so they must be included in our diets.

Atherosclerosis

Atherosclerosis, also known as 'hardening of the arteries', is a condition in which the wall of an artery thickens as a result of a build-up of fatty materials such as cholesterol.

Cholesterol

Cholesterol is a soft, waxy substance found among the fats (lipids) in the bloodstream and in all cells in the body. It is an important part of a healthy body because it is used to form cell membranes, some hormones and is needed for other functions. But a high level of cholesterol in the blood is a major risk for heart disease, which leads to heart attack.

Cholesterol and other fats cannot dissolve in the blood. They have to be transported to and from the cells by special carriers known as lipoproteins. There are several kinds, but the ones to focus on are low-density lipoprotein (LDL) and high-density lipoprotein (HDL).

LDL Cholesterol

Low-density lipoprotein is the major cholesterol carrier in the blood. If too much LDL cholesterol circulates in the blood, it can slowly build up in the walls of the arteries feeding the heart and brain. Together with other substances, it may form plaque that can clog those arteries. This condition is known as atherosclerosis. A clot that forms near this plaque can block the blood flow to part of the heart muscle and cause a heart attack. If a clot blocks the blood flow to part of the brain, it causes a stroke. That's why LDL cholesterol is known as 'bad' cholesterol. Lower levels of LDL cholesterol reflect a lower risk of heart disease.

HDL Cholesterol

High-density lipoprotein is a type of lipio found in the body. It serves a number of important functions, including scouring the blood for excess cholesterol, removing the excess to the liver, where it is broken down so that the body can eliminate it. This type of cholesterol is sometimes referred to as 'good cholesterol', because of its positive health benefits.

Free Radicals

Free radicals are atoms or groups of atoms with an unpaired number of electrons and can be formed when oxygen interacts with certain molecules. Once formed, these highly reactive radicals can start a chain reaction, like dominoes. Their main danger comes from the damage they can do when they react with important cellular components such as DNA or the cell membrane. Cells may function poorly or die if this occurs. To prevent free radical damage, the body has a defence system of antioxidants.

Glycemic Index

GI is a measure of the effects of carbohydrates on blood sugar levels. Carbohydrates that break down quickly during digestion and release glucose rapidly into the blood stream have a high GI; those that break down more slowly, releasing glucose more gradually, have a low GI.

Homocysteine

Homocysteine is an amino acid in the blood. Some studies have shown that too much homocysteine in the blood (plasma) is related to a higher risk of coronary heart disease and stroke.

Phytochemicals

Phytochemicals are non-nutritive plant chemicals that have protective or disease-preventive properties. There are more than a thousand known phytochemicals. It is well known that plants produce these chemicals to protect themselves but recent research demonstrates that they can protect humans against diseases too. Some of the well-known phytochemicals are lycopene in tomatoes, isoflavones in soya and flavonoids in fruits. These have all been mentioned in Chapter 1 on super foods.

Each phytochemical works differently. Here are some possible actions:

- Antioxidants – Most phytochemicals have antioxidant activity, protecting our cells against oxidative damage and reducing the risk of developing certain types of cancer. Phytochemicals with antioxidant activity include allyl sulfides (found in onions, leeks, garlic), carotenoids (fruits, carrots), flavonoids (fruits, vegetables) and polyphenols (tea, grapes).

- Hormonal action – Isoflavones, which are found in soya, imitate human oestrogens and help to reduce menopausal symptoms and osteoporosis.

- Stimulation of enzymes – Indoles, which are found in cabbage, stimulate enzymes that make oestrogen less effective and could reduce the risk of breast cancer. Other phytochemicals which interfere with enzymes are protease inhibitors (soya, beans) and terpenes (citrus fruits, cherries).

- Interference with DNA replication – Saponins, found in beans, interfere with the replication of cell DNA, thereby preventing the multiplication of cancer cells. Capsaicin, found in hot peppers, protects DNA from carcinogens.

- Anti-bacterial effect – The phytochemical, allicin, found in garlic, has anti-bacterial properties.

- Physical action – Some phytochemicals bind physically to cell walls thereby preventing the adhesion of pathogens to human cell walls. Proanthocyanidins are responsible for the anti-adhesion properties of cranberry. Consumption of cranberries will reduce the risk of urinary tract infections and will improve dental health.

Recipes

Some of these recipes are mine and some are from around the world. I found that some recipes are made differently in certain regions. That's not to say they don't taste good – having a variety of different cooking methods makes it more fun. I have adjusted some of the ingredients in the recipes to my own taste; you can do the same, but have fun with them. Enjoy!

Oven Temperature Conversions

This is an approximate conversion chart between gas mark and electric ovens. It should be accurate enough for all your cooking needs, though keep in mind that temperatures will vary between different types, brands and sizes of ovens, and also in relation to your location's altitude, temperature, humidity, etc.

Gas Mark	Fahrenheit	Celsius	Description
1/4	225	110	Very cool/Very slow
1/2	250	130	---
1	275	140	Cool
2	300	150	---
3	325	170	Very moderate
4	350	180	Moderate
5	375	190	---
6	400	200	Moderately hot
7	425	220	Hot
8	450	230	---
9	475	240	Very hot

Recipes

Chapter 7

Salads

I usually eat salads for lunch but you could serve any of these recipes as part of a dinner menu as a starter. If you eat any of the salads that contain fruit as a starter, wait at least 20 minutes after eating the salad, allowing time for it to be digested, before having your main meal.

Arabic Salad

This salad is simple, healthy and especially ideal for spring.

Serves 2

- ❑ 2 tomatoes, diced
- ❑ 1 courgette, peeled and chopped
- ❑ ½ red onion, finely chopped
- ❑ 1 tsp cumin
- ❑ 1 tsp coriander, finely chopped
- ❑ ½ tsp cayenne pepper
- ❑ 1 lemon, juiced
- ❑ 1 tbsp water
- ❑ 1 tbsp olive oil
- ❑ 1 tsp flaxseed oil
- ❑ ½ tsp sesame oil
- ❑ Parsley to serve

1. Add the tomatoes, courgette and onion in a salad bowl.
2. Mix the spices, lemon juice, water and oils together and pour over the vegetables.
3. Toss and refrigerate for 1 hour. Serve with a few sprigs of parsley.

Cucumber Salad

A cool, refreshing salad recipe – delicious any time of the year.

Serves 2–4

- ❑ 2 medium cucumbers
- ❑ 1 red onion
- ❑ 1 tomato, chopped
- ❑ 5 sprigs of parsley, chopped
- ❑ 2 tbsp fresh basil
- ❑ 2 tbsp fresh mint
- ❑ 1 tsp flaxseed oil
- ❑ 1 tbsp olive oil
- ❑ 1 garlic clove, minced
- ❑ 1 tbsp balsamic vinegar

1. Slice the cucumbers and onion thinly and place in a bowl. Add the chopped tomato and parsley.
2. Chop the basil and mint and toss them in.
3. Mix the oils, garlic and vinegar. Pour over the cucumber and toss together. Refrigerate for 1 hour and serve.

Salads

Fruited Rice Salad on Avocado Halves

The flavours of the rice, raisins, apricots and avocado tossed with the dressing makes this salad taste just exquisite.

Serves 4

❑ 225 g brown rice
❑ 5 mm fresh ginger, finely chopped
❑ 285 ml water
❑ 3 tbsp white wine (add a bit more if required!)
❑ 50 g raisins
❑ 50 g dried apricots, chopped
❑ 50 g almonds, chopped
❑ 2 avocados

Dressing
❑ 2 tbsp olive oil
❑ 1 tbsp flaxseed oil
❑ 1 lime, juiced
❑ 1 tsp balsamic vinegar
❑ 1 tsp maple syrup
❑ ¼ tsp curry powder
❑ ¼ tsp dry mustard

1. Mix all the dressing ingredients together and set aside.
2. Put the rice, ginger and water in a small saucepan and boil for 15 minutes or until the rice is just cooked.
3. Add the wine. Cover tightly and simmer for 10 minutes on a low heat.
4. Add the raisins, apricots and almonds. Cover and let sit with the heat off for 15 minutes.
5. Mix in the dressing and refrigerate for 1 hour.
6. Just before serving, halve, seed and peel the avocados. Fill each half with the rice salad. Spoon extra rice salad onto each plate and set the avocado half in it.

Grapefruit and Avocado Salad

This versatile salad combines classic flavours with a fresh twist. I occasionally use an orange instead of the grapefruit – it's still yummy!

Serves 2

❑ 1 grapefruit
❑ 1 small red onion, finely chopped
❑ 1 tbsp dill, chopped
❑ 1 tbsp olive oil
❑ 1 tsp flaxseed oil
❑ 1 lime, juiced
❑ 1 head romaine lettuce
❑ 1 ripe avocado

1. Section the grapefruit into a salad bowl with the chopped onion, dill, oils and lime juice. Refrigerate for 1 hour.
2. Chop the lettuce into bite-sized pieces, cube the avocado and add to the grapefruit mix just before serving.

Mixed Vegetable Salad

I sometimes add a teaspoon of honey to the dressing to give the salad a bit of a twist.

Serves 2–4

- ❏ 1 head broccoli, chopped into florets
- ❏ 1 head cauliflower, chopped
- ❏ 2 carrots, sliced
- ❏ 1 red onion, chopped
- ❏ 1 (200g) bag bean sprouts (mung bean or mixed)
- ❏ Bok choy, chopped
- ❏ 1 red bell pepper, chopped
- ❏ 50g raisins

Health dressing
- ❏ 1 clove garlic
- ❏ ¼ tsp mustard (optional)
- ❏ ¼ tsp parsley stalks, finely chopped
- ❏ 1 tbsp extra virgin olive oil
- ❏ 1 tsp flaxseed oil
- ❏ 1 tsp balsamic vinegar

1. Crush the garlic, mustard and parsley together, and then mix with the liquid ingredients.
2. Place all the vegetables and raisins in a salad bowl and toss with the health dressing.

Salat Katzutz
(Chopped Salad – Israeli Salad)

This is a signature dish, used mostly in Israeli breakfasts. The vegetables should be as fresh as possible.

Serves 4

- ❏ 1 cucumber, chopped
- ❏ 2 firm and ripe tomatoes, chopped
- ❏ ½ red onion, finely chopped
- ❏ ½ red bell pepper, chopped (optional)
- ❏ 4 sprigs of parsley, chopped

Dressing
- ❏ 1 tbsp olive oil
- ❏ 1 lemon, juiced
- ❏ Salt and pepper

1. Put the chopped vegetables in a salad bowl. Peel the cucumber before chopping if it is not organic, but this is not essential. Chop the onion slightly finer than the other vegetables.
2. For the dressing, mix the olive oil, lemon juice, salt and pepper together and pour over the vegetables. Toss and refrigerate.

African Fruit Salad

This combination of greens and fruit is served in all parts of Africa.

Serves 4

- ❏ 200g spinach (preferably baby spinach)
- ❏ 2 heads romaine lettuce
- ❏ 1 head lettuce
- ❏ 1 fresh pineapple, cut into fingers
- ❏ 2 fresh mangos, cut into strips
- ❏ 1 fresh coconut, cut into strips
- ❏ 1 orange, cut into strips with the skin left on
- ❏ 2 avocados, cut into strips and dipped in lemon
- ❏ 1 lemon, juiced
- ❏ 2 bananas, cut into chunks
- ❏ 2 tbsp hazelnuts, chopped
- ❏ 225g strawberries, halved
- ❏ 3 limes, zested and juiced
- ❏ 280ml mayonnaise
- ❏ 150ml whipped cream
- ❏ 2 tbsp honey or agave nectar

1. Stem, wash and tear into medium-sized pieces all the greens and place in a salad bowl.
2. Cut the pineapple into fingers and the mangos, coconut and orange into strips, leaving the skin on the orange. Cut the avocados into strips and dip them in lemon juice. Cut the bananas into chunks, dip them in mayonnaise and coat with chopped hazelnuts. Cut the strawberries in half.
3. Grate the limes and add the rinds and lime juice to the mayonnaise, cream and honey or agave nectar.
4. Mix the fruit together with the greens and serve.

Mango Salad

Serves 4–6

- ❏ 2 mangos
- ❏ ½ fresh pineapple
- ❏ 1 orange, juiced
- ❏ 1 lemon, juiced
- ❏ 4 avocados (optional)
- ❏ 225g strawberries

1. Cut the mangos and pineapple into 1 cm cubes and place in a bowl.
2. Mix the orange and lemon juice together and pour over the mango and pineapple.
3. Peel, seed and halve the avocados. Place on plates and scoop fruit into each half.
4. Garnish with strawberries and serve.

Peri-Peri Chicken or Turkey and Prawn Mango Salad (Nigerian)

I tried this for the first time at a friend's dinner party and I just had to include it in this book.

....

Serves 4

- ❑ 2 (200 g) chicken breasts (or turkey)
- ❑ 225 g large king prawns
- ❑ Peri-peri sauce
- ❑ 2 large mangos, firm and ripe
- ❑ 2 large avocados, firm and ripe
- ❑ 2 sweet red peppers (pimento)
- ❑ 200 g cherry tomatoes
- ❑ Rocket salad
- ❑ ½ red onion

Dressing
- ❑ 2 tbsp olive oil
- ❑ 1 lime, juiced
- ❑ 1 bunch coriander, chopped
- ❑ Salt and pepper to taste

1. Cut the chicken into strips.
2. Marinate the chicken and prawns in peri peri sauce.
3. Sauté the prawns until cooked.
4. Grill or bake the chicken until cooked through, then set aside to cool.
5. Cut the mangos and avocados into strips. Chop the red peppers and cut the tomatoes in half.
6. Wash the rocket leaves and place in a bowl. Add all the other ingredients.
7. Mix the olive oil, lime juice, coriander, salt and pepper. Pour over the salad and toss.

Salads

Thai Tuna or Chicken Fruit Salad

This salad is great with either tuna or chicken. If your tastebuds cannot handle chilli, use less or leave it out altogether.

Serves 4

- ❑ 8 lettuce leaves (use different kinds)
- ❑ 2 tbsp coriander, chopped
- ❑ 2 tbsp fresh mint, chopped
- ❑ 1 orange, peeled and sectioned
- ❑ 1 can tuna or 1 chicken breast, cooked and shredded
- ❑ 225 g red seedless grapes, halved
- ❑ ½ cucumber, sliced
- ❑ 1 small red onion, thinly sliced

Dressing
- ❑ Zest of 1 lime
- ❑ Juice of 2 limes
- ❑ 3 garlic cloves
- ❑ 2 serrano chillies, halved, seeded and cut into pieces
- ❑ 1½ tbsp fish or soy sauce
- ❑ 1 tbsp honey or agave nectar
- ❑ 5 tbsp cashews, chopped

1. Place half the lettuce in a bowl or on a platter. Tear the rest of the lettuce leaves into bite sizes and add to the bowl or platter.
2. Sprinkle the coriander and mint over the lettuce leaves.
3. Add the orange, tuna or chicken, grapes, cucumber and red onion. Refrigerate this while you make the dressing.
4. Grate the lime zest into a blender or food processor. Add the garlic, chillies, lime juice, fish or soy sauce and honey or agave, and blend until smooth.
5. Pour the dressing over the salad. Garnish with cashews and serve.

Indonesian Rice Salad

Adjust the sweetness of the dressing to your own personal taste.

Serves 4–6

- ❑ 250 g brown rice, cooked
- ❑ 5 tbsp peanut oil
- ❑ 3 tbsp sesame oil
- ❑ 1 orange, juiced
- ❑ 1 garlic clove
- ❑ ¼ tsp cayenne pepper
- ❑ 2 tbsp soy sauce
- ❑ 1 tsp salt
- ❑ 2 tbsp apple cider vinegar
- ❑ 1 can pineapple, crushed
- ❑ 3 spring onions, chopped
- ❑ 1 celery stalk, chopped
- ❑ 110 g bean sprouts
- ❑ 110 g raisins
- ❑ 110 g peanuts, chopped
- ❑ 110 g cashew pieces
- ❑ 2 tbsp sesame seeds
- ❑ 1 green pepper, chopped
- ❑ 1 red pepper, chopped
- ❑ 225 g water chestnut, minced

1. Put the cooked rice in a large bowl.
2. Add the oils, orange juice, garlic, cayenne pepper, soy sauce, salt, vinegar and pineapple and mix well.
3. Mix in the spring onions, celery, sprouts, raisins, peanuts, cashews, sesame seeds, peppers and water chestnuts.
4. Refrigerate for 1 hour, allowing the salad to chill and marinate.

Sesame-Spinach Salad
(Shigmchi Namul – Korean)

Use this salad as an accompaniment to grilled chicken or fish.

Serves 2–4

❑ 200 g bag of spinach
❑ 1 litre water

Dressing
❑ ¼ tsp salt (optional)
❑ ½ tsp honey or agave nectar
❑ 1 tsp soy sauce
❑ 2 tbsp sesame oil
❑ 2 tsp sesame seeds

1. Wash the spinach and remove the stems.
2. Bring the water with a little salt to a boil. Blanch the spinach in the hot water and then remove to an ice water bath.
3. Drain the spinach when cool and squeeze it by hand to remove excess moisture. Transfer to a cutting board and chop with a knife.
4. Mix the salt, honey or agave nectar, soy sauce and sesame oil in a bowl, and set aside.
5. Toss the spinach and dressing in a bowl and garnish with sesame seeds.

Asian Twisted Rice Salad

A nutritious Asian salad that can be served hot or cold.

Serves 4

❑ 250 g brown or Thai rice, cooked
❑ 1 carrot, chopped or shredded
❑ 2 spring onions
❑ 2 celery stalks, chopped
❑ 1 apple, cored and chopped
❑ 110 g Chinese peas cut horizontally into 1 cm pieces
❑ 50 g peanuts, chopped

Dressing
❑ 8 tbsp olive oil
❑ 2 tbsp soy sauce
❑ 1 lemon or lime, juiced
❑ 1 tsp dark sesame oil
❑ 1 garlic clove, crushed

1. Put all the vegetables and fruit in a salad bowl and toss with the cooked rice.
2. Sprinkle with half the nuts, leaving the rest for garnishing.
3. Whisk the olive oil, soy sauce, lemon juice, sesame oil and garlic in a small bowl.
4. Add half the dressing to the salad and taste. You might require more dressing depending on the type of rice used.
5. Garnish with the remaining nuts.

Salads

Indian Tomato Salad

The dressing for this salad gives a divine taste of India.

Serves 2

- ❑ 4 tbsp olive or grapeseed oil
- ❑ 2 tbsp wine vinegar
- ❑ 1 lime, juiced
- ❑ 1 garlic clove, crushed
- ❑ 1 tsp Dijon mustard
- ❑ ¼ tsp ground cumin
- ❑ ¼ tsp salt
- ❑ ¼ tsp ground black pepper
- ❑ 5 sprigs fresh mint, chopped
- ❑ 2 large tomatoes, sliced
- ❑ 1 red onion, thinly sliced
- ❑ ½ cucumber, thinly sliced

1. In a large bowl, whisk together the oil, vinegar, lime juice, garlic, mustard, cumin, salt and pepper.
2. Stir in the mint. Add the tomatoes, onion, and cucumber, and toss gently.
3. Garnish with additional mint leaves. Cover and refrigerate for up to 2 hours.
4. Serve as a side dish with any meal. It goes very well with chicken or salmon.

Greek Salad

Greek salad is a salad bar staple. When it is prepared with proper ingredients it encompasses everything that is good about the simple food of the Mediterranean.

Serves 2

- ❑ 1 head romaine lettuce, torn into bite-sized pieces
- ❑ 1 red onion, sliced
- ❑ 1 cucumber, sliced
- ❑ 4 tomatoes, sliced
- ❑ Kalamata olives
- ❑ Feta cheese, crumbled

Dressing
- ❑ 4 tbsp olive oil
- ❑ 1 lemon, juiced
- ❑ 2 garlic cloves, crushed
- ❑ 1 tsp dried oregano

1. Whisk together the oil, lemon, garlic and oregano, and set aside.
2. Put all the vegetables in a bowl. Add the olives and cheese.
3. Pour the dressing over the salad and toss.
4. Serve with pita and humous.

Apple and Spinach Salad

I prefer to use gala apples for this, but any type of apple is fine except Granny Smith's.

Serves 2

- ❏ 3 apples, peeled, cored and diced
- ❏ 3 spring onions, chopped
- ❏ 3 celery stalks, chopped
- ❏ 2 lemons, juiced
- ❏ 4 tbsp mayonnaise
- ❏ 4 tbsp tahini
- ❏ 2 tbsp honey or agave nectar
- ❏ 1 bunch spinach, torn into bite-sized pieces (or 1 100 g bag)
- ❏ 4 tbsp sesame seeds

1. Put the apples, onions and celery in a large bowl. Sprinkle with the juice of 1 lemon to avoid discolouration, and set aside.
2. In a blender or bowl, blend or whisk the mayonnaise, tahini, honey or agave and the remaining lemon juice until the mixture thickens.
3. Mix into the salad. Cover and refrigerate until it is time to serve.
4. Just before serving, toss in the spinach and garnish with sesame seeds.

Greek Sweet Potato Salad

Use an additional lemon if required.

Serves 2–4

- ❏ 4 sweet potatoes
- ❏ 1 red onion, sliced
- ❏ 4 tbsp olive oil
- ❏ 1 lemon, juiced
- ❏ 2 celery stalks, chopped
- ❏ Salt and black pepper to taste
- ❏ 5 sprigs parsley, chopped

1. Boil the potatoes until tender and keep them hot.
2. Place the onion in a large bowl. Sprinkle with salt and cold water and allow to stand for 5 minutes. Then drain.
3. Slice the potatoes and add to the onions. Add the olive oil, lemon juice and celery, and mix well to absorb the dressing.
4. Season with salt and pepper and garnish with parsley. Serve warm.

Mechouia
(Grilled Vegetable Salad – Tunisian)

This traditional Tunisian recipe combines grilled vegetables and hot chilli to make a delicious salad. This recipe is ideal for barbecues.

Serves 2

- ❑ 2 large red bell peppers
- ❑ 4 medium tomatoes
- ❑ 2 large red onions
- ❑ 1 small hot pepper
- ❑ 1 can tuna
- ❑ 4 tbsp feta cheese, crumbled

Dressing
- ❑ 3 tbsp olive oil
- ❑ 1 lemon, juiced
- ❑ 1 tsp oregano
- ❑ Salt and black pepper to taste

1. Grill the peppers, tomatoes and onions in a hot oven at 200°C. Turn over once and grill until soft. Remove from the oven and cool.
2. Remove the seeds from the pepper and chop all the vegetables into small pieces.
3. Place the vegetables on a serving platter and top with tuna and feta cheese.
4. Whisk the olive oil, lemon juice, oregano, salt and pepper, and pour over the salad. Serve.

Macedonian Salad

I know cabbage is not everyone's favourite vegetable but think of the nutritional benefits and vitamins.

Serves 4

- ❑ ¼ head white cabbage
- ❑ ⅛ head red cabbage
- ❑ 1 green pepper, chopped
- ❑ 1 red pepper, chopped
- ❑ 4 sprigs parsley, chopped
- ❑ 2 celery stalks, chopped
- ❑ 1 carrot
- ❑ 2 tbsp olive oil
- ❑ ½ lemon, juiced
- ❑ Salt to taste

1. Cut the cabbage into thin strips and place in a bowl.
2. Add the peppers, parsley and celery.
3. Grate the carrot and add to the bowl.
4. Sprinkle with olive oil, lemon juice and salt to taste. Mix well and serve.

Salads

Vegetable and Pomegranate Salad

Pomegranate makes this salad more interesting and adds a bit of a twist for your taste buds.

Serves 2–4

- ❑ 2 green bell peppers, cut into 1 cm cubes
- ❑ 4 large tomatoes, cut into 1 cm cubes
- ❑ 2 red onions, chopped finely
- ❑ 2 cucumbers, peeled and cut into 1 cm cubes
- ❑ ½ pomegranate

Dressing
- ❑ 4 tbsp olive oil
- ❑ 2 tbsp white wine vinegar
- ❑ ¼ tsp coarse salt and black pepper

1. Put the vegetables in a bowl.
2. Mix the olive oil, vinegar, salt and pepper together. Add the dressing to the salad and toss.
3. Hold the pomegranate over the salad. Using a spatula or spoon, release the seeds and juice over the salad.
4. Refrigerate for 1 hour before serving.

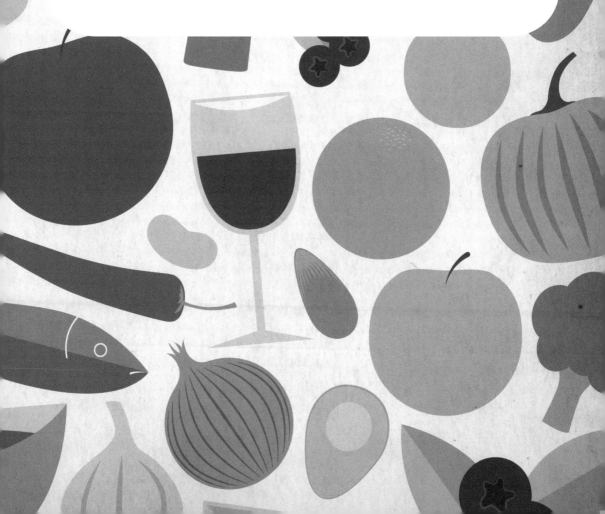

Chapter 8

Dressings and Dips

It is easy to make your own dressings and dips, try to be creative – adjust the ingredients in this section to your own taste. Just think, you are making your own dressings that contain absolutely no preservatives, how fabulous is that!

Salad Dressings

Healthy Dressing

....

- ❑ 1 tbsp extra virgin olive oil
- ❑ 1 tsp flaxseed oil
- ❑ 1 tsp balsamic vinegar
- ❑ 1 garlic clove
- ❑ ¼ tsp dry mustard
- ❑ ¼ tsp parsley, finely chopped

Mash the garlic, mustard and parsley together. Mix with other ingredients. Use this dressing with any salad.

Lemon Mint Dressing

....

- ❑ 4 tbsp fresh mint, chopped
- ❑ 4 tbsp fresh parsley, chopped
- ❑ 1 lemon
- ❑ 2 tbsp olive oil
- ❑ 1 tsp flaxseed oil

Mix all ingredients together and use over salad. Try it with cucumber salad.

Asian Dressing

....

- ❑ 1 lime
- ❑ 3 garlic cloves
- ❑ 2 serrano chillies, halved, seeded and chopped
- ❑ 1½ tbsp fish sauce or soy sauce
- ❑ 1 tbsp honey or agave nectar

Crush the garlic and mix in with all other ingredients.

Indian Style Dressing

- ❑ 4 tbsp grapeseed oil
- ❑ 2 tbsp white wine vinegar
- ❑ Juice of ½ fresh lime
- ❑ 1 garlic clove
- ❑ 1 tsp Dijon mustard
- ❑ ¼ tsp ground cumin
- ❑ ¼ tsp salt
- ❑ ¼ tsp ground black pepper
- ❑ 2 tbsp mint, chopped

Crush the garlic with the mint and mix in with the other ingredients.

Greek Dressing

- ❑ 3 tbsp olive oil
- ❑ 1½ tbsp red or white-wine vinegar
- ❑ ½ tsp salt
- ❑ ¼ tsp oregano
- ❑ ¼ tsp freshly-ground black pepper

Put all ingredients in a small jar, close and shake thoroughly. Chill before serving.

Sicilian Dressing

- ❑ 4 tbsp extra virgin olive oil
- ❑ 2 tbsp red-wine vinegar
- ❑ 80ml water
- ❑ ½ tsp salt
- ❑ ½ tsp black pepper
- ❑ 1 tsp oregano
- ❑ 1 tsp garlic powder or 1 garlic clove, crushed

Put all ingredients in a jar and shake thoroughly.

Dips

Red Pepper Dip

- ❑ 3 red peppers
- ❑ 2 tbsp fresh lemon juice
- ❑ 2 tbsp fresh parsley
- ❑ 1 tbsp olive oil
- ❑ Salt to taste

1. Cut and deseed the red peppers.
2. Bake them in the oven on a low temperature for about 20–25 minutes. Then remove the skin.
3. In a food processor, blend the peppers, lemon juice, parsley, olive oil and salt.
4. Serve with any veggie sticks such as carrots or cucumbers.

Salsa Dip

- ❑ 5 tomatoes, chopped
- ❑ 1 jalapeno pepper, chopped
- ❑ 1 red bell pepper, chopped
- ❑ 2 tbsp coriander, finely chopped
- ❑ 2 tbsp parsley, finely chopped
- ❑ 1 small red onion, finely chopped
- ❑ 2 garlic cloves, crushed
- ❑ 1 tsp balsamic vinegar or lemon juice

Mix all ingredients together, chill and serve.

Yellow Split Pea Dip

- ❑ 250g dried yellow split peas, rinsed and drained
- ❑ ¾ tsp salt
- ❑ ½ tsp black pepper
- ❑ 1 litre water
- ❑ 1 onion, chopped
- ❑ 2 tbsp extra virgin oil
- ❑ 1 tomato, finely chopped
- ❑ 1 red bell pepper, finely chopped
- ❑ 1 tbsp fresh parsley, chopped

1. Put the split peas with a pinch of salt and black pepper in a saucepan. Pour in enough water to cover the peas by 2½ cm and bring to the boil. Reduce the heat to medium and simmer, uncovered, stirring occasionally and adding more water, a little at a time, if it gets too thick before the peas get soft which takes about an hour.
2. Mash the peas and allow to cool.
3. Stir in half the onion, oil and remaining salt and pepper. Spread this purée out in a shallow bowl.
4. In a small bowl, mix the remaining onion, tomato, red pepper and parsley. Sprinkle over the purée.

Dressings and Dips

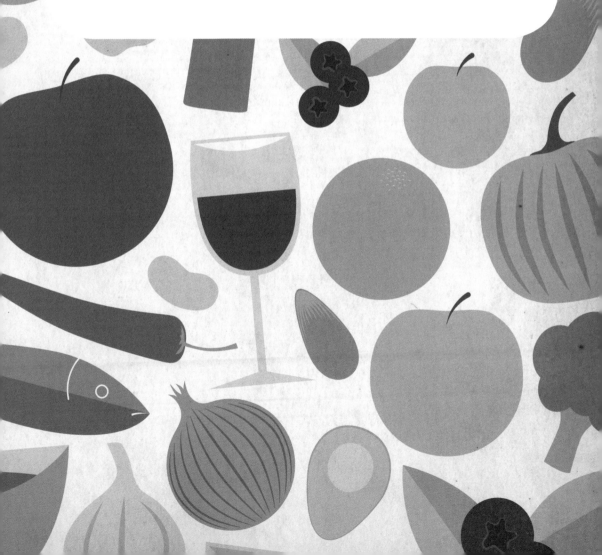

Chapter 9

Soups

Soups are very nutritious and
warming, especially during winter.

Mixed Vegetable Soup

This is a delightful and nutritious winter warmer, but it's also great at any time.

Serves 2–4

- ❑ 1 tbsp olive oil
- ❑ 2½ cm ginger, crushed
- ❑ 1 garlic clove, crushed
- ❑ 2 carrots, finely chopped
- ❑ 1 head cauliflower, chopped
- ❑ 50g broccoli, chopped
- ❑ 1 red pepper, chopped
- ❑ ½ head cabbage, finely chopped
- ❑ 5 green beans, chopped
- ❑ 600 ml water
- ❑ 2 potatoes, chopped
- ❑ ½ tsp soy sauce
- ❑ ¼ tsp red chilli powder
- ❑ 1 medium onion, chopped
- ❑ ½ tsp honey or agave nectar

1. Heat the oil in a saucepan. Add the ginger and garlic, and cook for 1 minute.
2. Add all the vegetables except the potatoes and onion.
3. Add salt and stir-fry for 4–5 minutes or until the vegetables are cooked.
4. Pour in the water and bring to the boil.
5. Add the potatoes, soy sauce and chilli. Boil until the soup becomes thick and transparent.
6. Finally, add the chopped onion and honey or agave nectar and boil for another 2–3 minutes. Serve hot.

Saffron-rich Soup
(Middle Eastern)

This soup is full of interesting combinations of flavours. Saffron is an expensive and rich golden spice, which has several health benefits such as improving blood circulation and anti-cancer and antioxidant properties.

Serves 4–6

- ❑ 4 tbsp olive oil
- ❑ 2 medium onions, chopped
- ❑ 2 fennel bulbs, chopped
- ❑ 3 garlic cloves, crushed
- ❑ 1 tsp saffron
- ❑ 1 tbsp boiling water
- ❑ 125 ml white wine
- ❑ 50 g fresh basil, shredded
- ❑ 1 kg tomatoes, finely chopped
- ❑ 450 ml water
- ❑ Salt and black pepper to taste
- ❑ 100g shredded basil to garnish

1. Heat the oil in a large pot. Sauté the onions, fennel and garlic over a medium heat for about 10 minutes.
2. Crumble and soak the saffron in 1 tbsp of boiling water for 5 minutes.
3. Pour the wine and soaked saffron, into the onions, fennel and garlic, then stir in 50 g of basil. Bring to a boil, then reduce the heat and simmer for a minute or two.
4. Add the chopped tomatoes and water. Bring to a boil, reduce the heat and simmer for about 30 minutes, partially covered.
5. Before serving, add salt and black pepper to taste, then stir in the basil. Serve hot.

Shrimp Soup (Portuguese)

Packed full of vegetables and flavour, this soup can be served as a substantial first course. By adding some more shrimps, you have a whole meal. I prefer to use jumbo shrimps.

Serves 4

- ❑ 2 tbsp olive oil
- ❑ 1 onion, coarsely chopped
- ❑ 2 garlic cloves, crushed
- ❑ 2 cans of tomatoes, deseeded and chopped, reserving juice
- ❑ 4 portobello mushrooms, sliced
- ❑ 5 parsley sprigs, chopped
- ❑ 2 celery stalks, chopped
- ❑ 1 bay leaf
- ❑ ½ tsp black pepper
- ❑ ½ tsp cayenne pepper
- ❑ 1 litre fish stock
- ❑ 200 ml dry white wine
- ❑ 2 potatoes
- ❑ 450g raw shrimps, peeled
- ❑ ½ tsp salt

1. In a large saucepan, sauté the onion and garlic in oil for about 5 minutes.
2. Mix in the tomatoes, mushrooms, parsley, celery, bay leaf, black pepper and cayenne pepper. Lower the heat and cook for about 10–15 minutes.
3. Slowly pour in the fish stock and wine. Stir through and bring to the boil.
4. When the soup is boiling, grate in the potatoes and allow the mixture to thicken. Reduce the heat and stir in the peeled shrimps. Simmer for 10–15 minutes.
5. Add salt to taste and serve.

Fish Soup with Orzo
(Italian)

Guaranteed to satisfy the most demanding of seafood lovers, this Italian version of fish soup is not only filling but wholesome as well.

• •

Serves 4–6

- ❑ 2 garlic cloves, sliced
- ❑ 1 tsp cumin
- ❑ 1 tsp paprika
- ❑ ½ tsp salt
- ❑ ½ tsp black pepper
- ❑ 4 tbsp tomato purée
- ❑ 2 tbsp olive oil
- ❑ 1 medium onion, thinly sliced
- ❑ 1 litre fish stock
- ❑ 450g sea bass cut in chunks
- ❑ 200g shrimps
- ❑ 75g orzo (rice-shaped pasta or any other soup pasta – add more if required)
- ❑ 4 parsley sprigs, chopped
- ❑ ½ each of lemon and lime, sliced thinly

1. Crush the garlic with the cumin, paprika, salt and pepper in a food processor. Then mix in the tomato purée.
2. Heat the oil in a large saucepan. Add the onion and sauté for about 5 minutes.
3. Add the spice mixture and stir for 3 minutes.
4. Pour in the fish stock and bring to the boil. Lower the heat and add the fish and shrimps. Cook for 10 minutes.
5. Add the orzo and cook for 10 minutes.
6. Garnish with parsley and serve with wedges of lime and lemon on the side.

Shiitake Bok Choy Soup
(Asian)

Chicken can be added to this recipe if desired. If so, use a diced chicken breast and boil together with the carrots and mushrooms.

Serves 4

- ❑ ½ onion, chopped
- ❑ 2 carrots, peeled and sliced
- ❑ 10 dried shiitake mushrooms, broken up
- ❑ 700 ml water
- ❑ 2 tbsp sesame oil
- ❑ 1 tsp honey or agave nectar
- ❑ 1 cm ginger, crushed
- ❑ 1 tbsp soy sauce
- ❑ ½ tsp each salt and black pepper
- ❑ 110 g bok choy

1. Put the onion, carrots and mushrooms into a saucepan and add the water. Bring to the boil and simmer until the carrots and mushrooms are soft.
2. Add the sesame oil, honey or agave, ginger and soy sauce. Add salt and black pepper to taste.
3. Bring back to the boil, then add the bok choy and simmer until it is tender which should take about 3 minutes.

Soups

Tomato Rasam Soup
(Indian)

In addition to the full spicy flavour, the best thing about this soup is that it does not require a lot of chopping! Leave out the red chilli peppers if you have a low tolerance to chilli.

Serves 2

- ❑ 5 tomatoes deseeded, 2 quartered and 3 chopped
- ❑ 1 garlic clove
- ❑ 550 ml water
- ❑ 2 tsp ginger, crushed
- ❑ 50g coriander, chopped
- ❑ 1 deseeded green chilli pepper, cut into small pieces
- ❑ 1 tsp curry powder
- ❑ ½ tsp cumin
- ❑ ½ tsp black pepper
- ❑ 2 tsp salt
- ❑ 2 tsp olive oil
- ❑ ¼ tsp black mustard seeds
- ❑ 2 deseeded red chilli peppers

1. Purée the quartered tomatoes with the garlic in a food processor and set aside.
2. Boil the water in a medium-sized saucepan. Add the puréed tomatoes, ginger, coriander and green chilli. Turn the heat down and simmer for 3 minutes.
3. Add the tomato and garlic purée, curry, cumin, black pepper and salt and simmer for 5 minutes.
4. Put the oil and mustard seed in a small saucepan over a high heat. Cover and cook until you hear the mustard seeds crackle, which takes about 1–2 minutes.
5. Add the red chillies and cook uncovered, stirring until they start to brown. This takes about 60 seconds. Pour into the soup and stir. Serve hot.

Soups

Spiced Tomato Soup (Indian)

This soup is deliciously spicy, completely vegetarian and has almost no cholesterol.

Serves 4

- ❑ 2 garlic cloves
- ❑ 1 serrano green chilli, seeded
- ❑ 1 onion, chopped coarsely
- ❑ 1 cucumber, diced
- ❑ 2 tbsp salt
- ❑ 450g tomatoes, firm and ripe
- ❑ 1 tbsp tamarind paste
- ❑ 225g fresh coriander, chopped
- ❑ 110g fresh mint, chopped
- ❑ 2½ cm ginger, grated
- ❑ 1 tsp ground cumin
- ❑ 225ml non-fat plain yoghurt (optional)
- ❑ 1 tsp olive oil
- ❑ 2 tsp cumin seeds
- ❑ 1 tsp yellow mustard seeds
- ❑ 1 tsp black mustard seeds

1. In a food processor, blend the garlic and chilli until minced. Add the onion and mince again. Scrape into a large bowl and stir in the cucumber and salt.
2. Meanwhile, bring 3 litres of water to the boil. Cut an X in the bottom of each tomato and immerse in the boiling water for 30 seconds or until the tomato skin begins to curl. Rinse under cold running water until cool and remove skins. Chop the tomatoes and add with the juice to the bowl containing the onion mixture.
3. In a small bowl, mix the tamarind paste with 4 tbsp of warm water and pour into the tomato mixture.
4. Add the coriander, mint and ginger, and mix.
5. In a saucepan over a medium heat, stir the cumin for 2 minutes, until fragrant.
6. Add the tomato mixture and 400 ml water, and bring to the boil. Remove from the heat, cover and chill for at least an hour.
7. Ladle the soup into bowls and top each serving with yoghurt (optional).
8. In a non-stick pan with a lid, add the oil, cumin and mustard seeds. Set over a high heat until the spices begin to pop.
9. Cover and shake vigorously until the popping subsides, which should take about 1–2 minutes. Spoon the hot seeds over the soup and serve.

Soups

Chicken Soba Soup with Spinach (Asian)

Soba is a thin Japanese noodle with a nutty flavour and delicate texture.

Serves 4–6

- ❑ 1 litre water
- ❑ 2 chicken breasts, cubed
- ❑ 2 tbsp grapeseed oil
- ❑ 300 g shiitake mushrooms, caps thinly sliced
- ❑ 4 spring onions, thinly sliced
- ❑ 1 garlic clove, crushed
- ❑ 2½ cm ginger, chopped
- ❑ ⅛ tsp salt (optional)
- ❑ 125 g soba noodles
- ❑ 1 bunch spinach, torn into bite sizes (or 100g bag)
- ❑ Juice of 1 lime
- ❑ 1 tbsp soy sauce
- ❑ Extra spring onions to serve, thinly sliced

1. In a large saucepan, add the water and chicken and boil for 15 minutes or until the chicken is cooked. Reserve the broth.
2. Heat the oil over a medium heat in a saucepan. Add the mushrooms, spring onions, garlic, ginger and season with salt. Stir occasionally until the mushrooms are cooked, which should take about 5 minutes.
3. Add the chicken broth to the mushroom mixture and bring to the boil. Add the soba noodles and chicken, reduce to a simmer and cook for about 5 minutes.
4. Add the spinach and cook until tender (about a minute). Add the lime juice and soy sauce.
5. Top with spring onions and serve.

Cream Soup
(Senegalese)

A creamy Senegalese soup with a strong curry flavour to it.

Serves 4

- ❑ 2 skinless chicken breasts, chopped (450 g)
- ❑ 1 litre water
- ❑ 2 tbsp olive oil-based or unsalted butter
- ❑ 3 Granny Smith apples, peeled, cored and chopped
- ❑ 2 celery stalks, chopped
- ❑ 2 carrots, chopped
- ❑ 1 onion, chopped
- ❑ 1 garlic clove, crushed
- ❑ 3 tbsp curry powder
- ❑ 50g golden raisins
- ❑ 1 sweet potato, diced
- ❑ 110 ml coconut milk
- ❑ Salt to taste
- ❑ ½ tsp cayenne
- ❑ ½ white pepper
- ❑ Mango chutney to garnish

1. Put the chicken in a large saucepan with 1 litres of water and bring to the boil.
2. Remove the chicken when cooked and set aside, reserving the broth.
3. In a saucepan, heat the oil-based fat or butter over a medium heat until the foam subsides.
4. Add the apples, celery, carrots, onion and garlic, stirring occasionally until they begin to soften which should take about 10 minutes.
5. Add the curry powder, chicken and raisins, and cook for about a minute. Add the diced sweet potato, cook and stir for 2 minutes.
6. Stir in the chicken broth, cover and simmer for 1 hour.
7. Stir in the coconut milk and salt to taste. Simmer uncovered for 10 minutes.
8. Add the cayenne and white pepper.
9. Cool the soup. Then pour into a food processor or blender in batches, and blend until smooth.
10. Strain the soup into a large bowl and chill for about 2 to 3 hours until cold.
11. Garnish with ½ teaspoon of chutney and serve.

Sweet Pea Soup
(East African)

I'm not a fan of peas but this turned out to be very delicious and nourishing.

Serves 4

- ❏ 2 onions, chopped
- ❏ 2 garlic cloves, crushed
- ❏ 2½ cm ginger, peeled and grated
- ❏ 1 tsp salt
- ❏ ¼ tsp cayenne pepper
- ❏ 1 tbsp garam masala
- ❏ 2 tomatoes, chopped
- ❏ 1 sweet potato, diced
- ❏ 700 ml water
- ❏ 600 g green peas

1. Sauté the onions and garlic in a saucepan for 5 to 10 minutes.
2. Add the ginger, salt, cayenne pepper and garam masala and cook for a few minutes, stirring often.
3. Mix in the tomatoes and sweet potato. Add 400 ml water and stir. Bring to the boil. Reduce the heat, cover and simmer for 5 minutes.
4. Add half the peas, cover and simmer for 10 minutes.
5. Remove from the heat and add the remaining water.
6. Blend in batches in a blender until smooth.
7. Return to the saucepan. Add the remaining peas and cook on a medium heat for 3–5 minutes.

Soups

Shorba
(Algerian)

Soup is typically the first course in an Algerian meal. This soup draws its flavours from a combination of spices, herbs and vegetables.

....

Serves 4–6

- ❏ 3 skinless chicken breasts, cubed
- ❏ 1 onion, grated
- ❏ ½ courgette, grated
- ❏ ½ potato, grated
- ❏ ½ celery stalk, chopped
- ❏ 1 carrot, chopped
- ❏ 2 tsp salt
- ❏ ½ tsp black pepper
- ❏ ½ tsp cinnamon
- ❏ 1 tbsp paprika
- ❏ 2 tbsp tomato paste
- ❏ 1 tbsp olive oil
- ❏ 50 g dried chick peas, soaked overnight in water and drained (or canned and drained is fine)
- ❏ 1 litre water
- ❏ 110 g orzo or other soup pasta
- ❏ 1 tbsp parsley, chopped
- ❏ 1 tsp fresh mint, chopped
- ❏ 1 lemon, sliced

1. Put the chicken, onion, courgette, potato, celery, carrot, salt, pepper, cinnamon, paprika, tomato paste, oil, chick peas (if using dried) and 700 ml water in a large pot.
2. Simmer covered over a low heat for 20 minutes.
3. Add the remaining water, bring to the boil and simmer for 45 minutes.
4. Add the orzo and chick peas (if using canned). Cook for 10 minutes.
5. Add the parsley and mint. Serve with lemon slices.

Soups

Fish Soup
(Cape Verdean)

*Cape Verdean food is an enticing mixture of Creole, Portuguese and African flavours.
The islands have a wealth of seafood, which is often cooked straight from the sea.
One of the national favourites is a slow-boiled stew of corn, beans, vegetables and
marinated tuna, called Catchupa.*

••

Serves 4

- ❑ 3 onions, chopped
- ❑ 4 spring onions, chopped
- ❑ 2 tomatoes, chopped
- ❑ 1 green bell pepper, chopped
- ❑ 1 red bell pepper, chopped
- ❑ 3 tbsp olive oil
- ❑ 1 kg sea bass or cod, cut into small pieces
- ❑ 1 litre water
- ❑ 6 potatoes, diced
- ❑ 3 sweet potatoes, diced
- ❑ 1 (30g) bunch fresh parsley, chopped

1. Sauté the chopped onions, spring onions, tomatoes and peppers in a large saucepan with the oil.
2. Add the cut fish and 1 litre of water and bring gently to the boil.
3. Add the potatoes and parsley. Reduce the heat and simmer. Add more potatoes if you want a thicker soup.

Soups

107

Vegetable Soup
(South African)

Every country has its own vegetable soup and South Africa is no exception. This soup should keep you warm in winter.

Serves 4–6

- ❑ 2 onions, chopped
- ❑ 1 garlic clove, crushed
- ❑ 30 ml olive oil
- ❑ 3 carrots, sliced
- ❑ 2 turnips, sliced
- ❑ 2 celery stalks, chopped
- ❑ 4 courgettes, sliced
- ❑ 1 small butternut squash, peeled, deseeded and chopped
- ❑ 2 medium brinjals/eggplants/ aubergines, peeled and diced
- ❑ 2 tbsp fresh tarragon or thyme, chopped
- ❑ 1 litre vegetable or chicken stock
- ❑ Salt and black pepper to taste

1. Sauté the onions and garlic in oil in a heavy-based saucepan for about 5 minutes.
2. Add the carrots, turnips, celery, courgettes, butternut squash, brinjals, tarragon or thyme and stock. Bring to the boil.
3. Reduce the heat, cover the saucepan and simmer for about 25 minutes or until the vegetables are soft.
4. Season to taste and serve.

Tomato and Carrot Soup

A nourishing soup, packed with vitamin C, beta-carotene and lycopene.

••

Serves 4–6

- ❑ 1 tbsp olive oil
- ❑ 1 onion, chopped
- ❑ 2 garlic cloves, chopped
- ❑ 2 carrots, peeled and chopped
- ❑ 500 g tomatoes, skinned and coarsely chopped
- ❑ 1 apple, peeled, cored and chopped
- ❑ 1 *bouquet garni*
- ❑ 1 bay leaf
- ❑ 1 litre vegetable or chicken stock
- ❑ Salt and freshly ground black pepper to taste
- ❑ 60 ml cream to garnish (optional)

1. Heat the oil in a large saucepan. Add the onion and garlic and sauté for 10 minutes.
2. Add the carrots and stir over a low heat until all the oil has been absorbed.
3. Add the tomatoes, apple, *bouquet garni*, bay leaf and stock.
4. Season with salt and black pepper, and bring to the boil. Cover the saucepan and simmer for 45 minutes.
5. Remove and discard the *bouquet garni*. Pour the soup into a blender.
6. Return the soup to the saucepan, heat through and adjust the seasoning.
7. Pour into individual bowls, garnish with 1 tbsp of cream (optional) and serve.

Soups

Sweet Potato Soup
(South African)

An extremely fibre-rich, spicy and satisfying soup. Use half the chilli or leave it out completely if you have a low tolerance to chilli.

Serves 4

- ❑ 1 tbsp olive oil
- ❑ 2 onions, chopped
- ❑ 1 serrano green chilli pepper or jalapeno, sliced thinly
- ❑ 1 litre vegetable or chicken stock
- ❑ 3 sweet potatoes, peeled and chopped
- ❑ 2½ cm ginger, grated
- ❑ 1 tsp thyme
- ❑ Salt and black pepper to taste
- ❑ 4 sausages, sliced thickly (optional)
- ❑ Juice of 1 lemon

1. Sauté the onions in the oil in a saucepan until transparent.
2. Add the sliced pepper and stock. Bring to the boil over a medium heat.
3. Add the sweet potatoes, ginger and thyme. Boil then reduce the heat and simmer for 25 minutes, stirring occasionally.
4. When the potatoes are cooked, pour into a food processor, solids first, and purée. Season with salt and black pepper to taste.
5. If you are having the soup hot and meaty, sauté the sausage separately until crisp. When ready to serve, stir in the lemon juice, then pour the soup into individual bowls, either cold or hot. Add the sausage, if applicable, and top with lemon curls.

Lentil and Courgette Soup
(Saudi Arabian)

This is a unique version of a traditional Saudi Arabian lentil soup. Serve with some warm pita bread for a thoroughly filling and nutritious meal.

Serves 4

- ❑ 275g dried lentils
- ❑ 1 onion, chopped
- ❑ 4 garlic cloves, crushed
- ❑ 1 litre water
- ❑ 2 potatoes, cut into small pieces
- ❑ 1 tsp cumin
- ❑ 1 celery stalk, chopped
- ❑ 2 courgettes, cut into small pieces
- ❑ Salt and black pepper to taste
- ❑ 2 lemons, cut into wedges to serve on the side

1. Put the lentils, onion and garlic into a large saucepan. Add the water, cover and bring to the boil. Reduce the heat and simmer for 20 minutes.
2. Stir in the potatoes, cumin, celery and courgettes. Cover and cook for 15 minutes, until the lentils and potatoes are tender.
3. Season with salt and black pepper to taste.
4. When the soup is ready to serve, pour it into soup bowls, sprinkle with lemon juice and serve a lemon wedge with each bowl.

Aromatic Carrot Soup
(Moroccan)

The mixture of spices, lemon and honey creates a burst of excitingly different flavours in this warming soup.

Serves 4

- ❑ 1 litre vegetable or chicken stock
- ❑ 450g carrots, peeled and chopped
- ❑ 1 garlic clove, crushed
- ❑ ⅛ tsp cinnamon
- ❑ ¼ tsp cumin
- ❑ ½ tsp paprika
- ❑ ½ tsp cayenne pepper or hot sauce
- ❑ Juice of 1 lemon
- ❑ ½ tsp honey or agave nectar
- ❑ ½ tsp orange flower water
- ❑ 1 tbsp parsley, chopped

1. In a medium saucepan, boil the stock. Add the carrots and garlic. Reduce the heat and simmer until the carrots are tender.
2. Remove half the carrots and set aside. In a food processor, blend the carrots, garlic and stock, then return to the saucepan.
3. Mix in the cinnamon, cumin, paprika and cayenne or hot sauce. Add the remaining carrots to the soup, and simmer for 10 minutes.
4. When the soup is ready to serve, stir in the lemon juice, honey or agave and orange flower water. Serve in bowls and sprinkle with parsley.

Chapter 10

Starters and Vegetables

Make sure you wash all vegetables thoroughly,
preferably in filtered or bottled water, especially if
veggies are not organic. I tend to wash veggies like
courgettes (veggies with skin) with salt or lemon.

Avocado Stuffed with Seafood
(South African)

If you love avocados, then this recipe will be a treat. It's an easy-to-prepare dish that can be served as a starter or snack at any time of the day.

Serves 2–4

- ❑ Juice of ½ lemon
- ❑ 4 tbsp dry white wine
- ❑ 1 tsp curry powder
- ❑ 150 g mayonnaise
- ❑ ½ tsp mace or nutmeg
- ❑ 225 g prawns, cleaned and deveined
- ❑ 450 g crabmeat or lobster meat
- ❑ 1 head romaine lettuce, cleaned and leaves separated
- ❑ 2 avocados, peeled and halved
- ❑ 1 grapefruit, peeled and sectioned

1. Mix the lemon juice, white wine, curry powder, mayonnaise and nutmeg in a small bowl and set aside.
2. Place the prawns and crabmeat in a bowl and add half the dressing. Leave to marinade slightly.
3. Arrange the lettuce leaves to form cups on plates. Place the avocado halves in the lettuce cups and spoon in the seafood and dressing. Place 4 grapefruit sections on the side of each plate and serve.

Asian-style Coleslaw

Crunchy, healthy coleslaw you can enjoy with any food or just on its own.

Serves 2–4

- ❑ ½ medium head white cabbage, sliced
- ❑ ½ medium head red cabbage, sliced
- ❑ 1 red pepper, chopped
- ❑ 1 yellow pepper, chopped
- ❑ 3 carrots, peeled and shredded
- ❑ 4 spring onions
- ❑ ½ bunch fresh coriander, chopped
- ❑ 50 g roasted peanuts, chopped
- ❑ 3 tbsp rice vinegar
- ❑ 1 tbsp sesame oil
- ❑ 2 tbsp soy sauce
- ❑ 1 tbsp honey or agave nectar
- ❑ 1 cm fresh ginger, peeled and minced
- ❑ 1 garlic clove, crushed
- ❑ 1 jalapeno pepper, deseeded and finely chopped

1. Toss the salad ingredients in a bowl.
2. Mix the vinegar, sesame oil, soy sauce, honey or agave, ginger, garlic and pepper. Mix into the salad.

Bean Cakes
(Moi-Moi – Nigerian)

A favourite side dish, especially at Nigerian parties. It is easy to prepare and quite healthy as the cooking method is steaming. You can get the peeled beans from the local African or Asian grocery stores. Banana leaves are usually used for cooking in cakes but, in their absence, I use the foil takeout boxes.

Serves 6

- ❑ 250g black-eyed beans (bean flour can be used but it's not the best option)
- ❑ 1 onion
- ❑ 1 red chilli pepper
- ❑ 2 tbsp dried ground crayfish
- ❑ 100 g cooked prawns
- ❑ 2 tbsp grapeseed oil
- ❑ 1 tsp salt
- ❑ 3 hard-boiled eggs (optional), cut into chunks
- ❑ 6 foil takeout boxes

Note. If using already peeled beans, just wash them thoroughly and blend.

1. Place the beans in a large bowl. Cover with water and soak overnight.
2. Rub the beans briskly between your palms to remove the skins. Fill the bowl with water and the skins will float to the top. Discard the skins. Continue this action until the beans are clean and no skins are left behind – soak them again if necessary.
3. In a food processor, blend the beans, onion, ground black pepper and 10 ml of water until smooth.
4. Pour into a bowl. Add the crayfish, prawns, oil and salt and mix thoroughly.
5. In a large saucepan, add enough water just to fill the base and bring to the boil. Use the foil boxes as a measuring guide: only half of the box should be submerged in water. Pour small amounts of the mixture into individual boxes. If you are using eggs, add some into each box. Cover with the lids, place in the saucepan and steam for an hour until firm.
6. Serve warm or hot with tomato sauce and salad.

Avocado with Peanut and Romaine Lettuce

Serves 4

- ❑ 3 avocados (ripe but firm), stone removed and cut into cubes
- ❑ Juice of ½ lemon
- ❑ 2 tbsp peanuts, ground
- ❑ ½ tsp cinnamon
- ❑ ½ tsp paprika
- ❑ Salt and chilli powder to taste
- ❑ 1 bunch romaine lettuce leaves, separated and washed
- ❑ 10 g fresh chives, chopped to garnish

1. Place the cubed avocado in a bowl and sprinkle with lemon juice. Set aside.
2. Mix the ground peanuts, cinnamon, paprika, salt and chilli powder together thoroughly.
3. Arrange the individual lettuce leaves on a platter like cups.
4. Scoop avocado onto each lettuce leaf, sprinkle peanut mixture over the avocado and garnish with chives.

Starters and Vegetables

Baked Sweet Potato Skins

Instead of the traditional potato skin, I use sweet potatoes for a slightly different twist.

Serves 4–6

- ❑ 3 large sweet potatoes
- ❑ 8 tbsp grated parmesan cheese
- ❑ 1 tbsp parsley, chopped
- ❑ 1 tsp basil, chopped
- ❑ ½ tsp garlic powder
- ❑ ½ tsp salt
- ❑ Olive oil spray
- ❑ 1 spring onion, finely chopped
- ❑ 110 ml fat-free sour cream

1. Preheat the oven to 200°C or Gas Mark 6.
2. Wash the potatoes thoroughly and pierce all over with a fork. Wrap them individually in foil and bake for an hour or until they are easily pierced with a fork. Remove and allow to cool slightly.
3. In a small bowl, mix the parmesan, parsley, basil, garlic powder and salt.
4. When the potatoes are cool enough to handle, quarter them length-wise. Scoop out the flesh, saving a ½ cm shell. Cut the strips in half crosswise – you should have 20–24 wedges.
5. Line a baking tray with foil. Place the wedges on the tray and coat lightly with olive oil spray. Top with the cheese mix.
6. Bake in the oven for about 10–12 minutes or until golden brown. Place on a serving platter, sprinkle with chopped spring onions and serve with sour cream.

Creamy Courgette and Garlic

A vegetarian dish everyone will love – it's nutritious as well.

∙∙∙

Serves 4–6

- ❑ 2 tbsp Olivio or unsalted butter
- ❑ 6 garlic cloves, crushed
- ❑ 1 onion, finely chopped
- ❑ 3 leeks, finely chopped
- ❑ 1 tsp fresh thyme, chopped
- ❑ 3 medium courgettes, washed and grated
- ❑ 3 medium yellow squash, washed and grated
- ❑ 2½ tbsp sour cream
- ❑ ½ tsp fresh ground black pepper

1. Melt the Olivio or butter in a saucepan. Add the garlic, onion and leeks and sauté over a low heat for 5 minutes.
2. Mix in the thyme, courgettes and squash. Cook, stirring frequently for 5–7 minutes or until the courgettes and squash are tender.
3. Place on a plate, top with sour cream and sprinkle with ground black pepper.

Bok Choy Slaw

A versatile side dish that goes well with lamb or chicken. Crunchy and absolutely delicious.

∙∙∙

Serves 4

- ❑ 4 tbsp rice wine vinegar
- ❑ 1 tbsp sesame oil
- ❑ 2 tsp honey
- ❑ 2 tsp Dijon mustard
- ❑ ¼ tsp salt
- ❑ 600 g bok choy, washed and thinly sliced
- ❑ 2 carrots, peeled and shredded
- ❑ 2 spring onions, chopped thinly

1. In a medium bowl, whisk the vinegar, oil, honey, mustard and salt until smooth.
2. Add the bok choy, carrots and spring onions.
3. Toss to coat thoroughly with the dressing.

Vegetable Stir Fry

An easy way of introducing vegetables as a side dish to your menu. You can make this dish sweet, spicy or have it as it is. Chicken or shrimps can be added to make it a meal on its own.

Serves 4

- ❏ 1 tbsp grapeseed oil
- ❏ 2 red onions, sliced
- ❏ 150 g mushrooms, sliced
- ❏ 2 courgettes, chopped
- ❏ 1 head white cabbage or Chinese cabbage, shredded
- ❏ 2 tbsp Szechuan stir-fry sauce
- ❏ 1 tsp sesame oil
- ❏ 1 tsp agave nectar or honey (optional)
- ❏ Salt and pepper to taste

1. Heat the grapeseed oil in a wok or saucepan. Sauté the onions for 2 minutes. Add the mushrooms and courgettes and cook for 3 minutes.
2. Mix in the cabbage. Drizzle the stir-fry sauce over the vegetables and sauté until the cabbage is just wilted.
3. Drizzle with sesame oil and agave or honey (if you are using it for a sweet twist). Add salt and pepper to taste. Mix thoroughly.

Spicy Vegetables

Serve this dish on its own or with wholemeal pitta bread.

Serves 2–4

- ❏ 2 tbsp olive oil
- ❏ 2 tsp black mustard seeds
- ❏ 2 onions, finely chopped
- ❏ 2 garlic cloves, chopped
- ❏ 1 cm ginger, chopped
- ❏ ½ tsp turmeric
- ❏ ½ tsp coriander
- ❏ 1 tsp ground cumin
- ❏ ¼ tsp chilli powder
- ❏ 2 carrots, peeled and chopped
- ❏ 2 sweet potatoes, peeled and chopped
- ❏ 2 tomatoes, chopped
- ❏ 250 g green beans, trimmed and cut into small pieces
- ❏ Salt and pepper to taste
- ❏ ½ tsp garam masala

1. Heat the oil in a heavy saucepan and fry the mustard seeds until they pop.
2. Add the onions, garlic and ginger. Sauté, stirring continuously for 5 minutes or until the onions are golden.
3. Add the turmeric, coriander, cumin and chilli powder, and sauté for about 30 seconds. Then toss in the vegetables. Mix until they are thoroughly coated with the spices.
4. Add salt, pepper and 3 tablespoons of water. Cover and cook for 15 minutes or until the vegetables are tender.
5. Stir gently every 5 minutes and add a little more water if necessary. Sprinkle with garam masala and stir.

Stewed Greens

This recipe is packed full of nutrients, vitamins, fibre, folic acid – you can't go wrong with it.

Serves 4–6

- ❑ 600 g collard greens, washed and chopped
- ❑ 200 g spinach, washed
- ❑ 200 g kale
- ❑ 4 tbsp olive oil
- ❑ 1 onion, chopped
- ❑ 4 tomatoes, chopped
- ❑ 1 green chilli pepper, deseeded and finely chopped
- ❑ Juice of ½ lemon
- ❑ 1 tbsp plain unbleached flour
- ❑ 225 ml water
- ❑ ½ tsp salt and black pepper

1. Steam the greens in a steamer for about 6 minutes. If you don't have a steamer, pour water into a saucepan and bring to the boil. Place the greens in a colander and insert into the saucepan. Cover and steam for about 6 minutes.
2. Heat 2 tbsp of oil in a frying pan over a medium heat. Add the onion, tomatoes and pepper. Mix well and cook for about 5 minutes. Reduce the heat to low and add the remaining oil.
3. Whisk the lemon juice, flour and half the water until smooth and well-blended. Pour into the onion mixture and mix well.
4. Add the remaining water, cooked greens, salt and pepper to taste and mix well. Increase the heat to medium, cover and cook for 3 minutes to heat through. Serve with a main dish such as fish or chicken.

Asparagus and Sun-dried Tomatoes

The combination of the sun-dried tomatoes and healthy sauce gives a wonderfully sweet and savoury taste. Serve this on its own as a starter or side dish with chicken or fish – absolutely delicious!

Serves 2

- ❏ 1 tbsp olive oil
- ❏ 1 tsp flaxseed oil
- ❏ 1 tsp balsamic vinegar
- ❏ ½ tsp cayenne pepper
- ❏ 2 tbsp sun-dried tomatoes, chopped
- ❏ 15 g parsley, chopped
- ❏ 225 g asparagus
- ❏ 10 g fresh basil, chopped

1. In a small bowl, mix the oils, vinegar, cayenne, tomatoes and half of the parsley together. Leave to marinade for 2 hours.
2. Steam the asparagus for about 6 minutes or until just tender.
3. Place the asparagus on a plate. Pour the sauce over, and sprinkle with the remaining parsley and basil.

Baked Tomatoes

A classic Mediterranean dish, which is often served as part of a number of platters making up a main meal.

Serves 2–4

- ❏ 2 tbsp olive oil
- ❏ 4 large tomatoes, cored and each cut into 3 thick slices
- ❏ 200 g breadcrumbs
- ❏ 20 g fresh basil, chopped
- ❏ 1 tsp fresh thyme, chopped
- ❏ 1 tsp fresh oregano, chopped
- ❏ 1 garlic clove, chopped
- ❏ Extra olive oil to drizzle

1. Preheat the oven to 180°C or Gas Mark 4.
2. Lightly brush half the olive oil on a baking tray. Arrange the tomato slices, cut side up, in a single layer.
3. Mix the breadcrumbs, remaining oil, half the herbs and garlic. Sprinkle over the tomatoes. Bake for about 5–7 minutes or until the breadcrumbs are lightly browned.
4. Place the tomatoes on a serving platter, sprinkle with remaining herbs and drizzle with olive oil.

Sautéed Bok Choy
(Asian)

Bok choy isn't just for salads or Asian dishes. It is also a perfect vegetable for a quick, healthy side dish. Sautéing concentrates both the flavour and nutrition of the vegetable.

Serves 2–4

- ❑ 1 onion, chopped
- ❑ 2½ cm ginger, grated
- ❑ 1 tbsp olive oil
- ❑ ½ tsp sesame oil
- ❑ 500 g bok choy, both white and green parts sliced
- ❑ 1 tbsp rice wine vinegar
- ❑ 1 tsp fish sauce
- ❑ ½ tsp red pepper, crushed
- ❑ Salt to taste
- ❑ 100 ml chicken stock
- ❑ 1 tbsp sesame seeds

1. In a medium-sized saucepan, sauté the onion and ginger in the oils for 5 minutes.
2. Add the bok choy, vinegar, fish sauce, pepper, salt and stock. Mix and sauté for about 8 minutes.
3. Place on a plate and sprinkle with sesame seeds.

Balsamic Mushrooms

These mushrooms can be served hot or cold, so you can prepare them a day before or right before you serve your main meal. They take 10 minutes to prepare.

Serves 2

- ❑ ½ tsp sesame oil
- ❑ 1 onion, chopped
- ❑ 350 g shiitake mushrooms
- ❑ 2 tbsp sundried tomatoes (optional)
- ❑ 2 tbsp balsamic vinegar
- ❑ 1 tbsp red wine
- ❑ 20 g parsley, chopped

1. Sauté the onion in sesame oil in a wok or saucepan for 5 minutes.
2. Add the mushrooms, sundried tomatoes, vinegar, red wine and half the parsley. Mix together thoroughly for 5 minutes, stirring continuously.
3. Place on a serving platter and sprinkle with the remaining parsley.

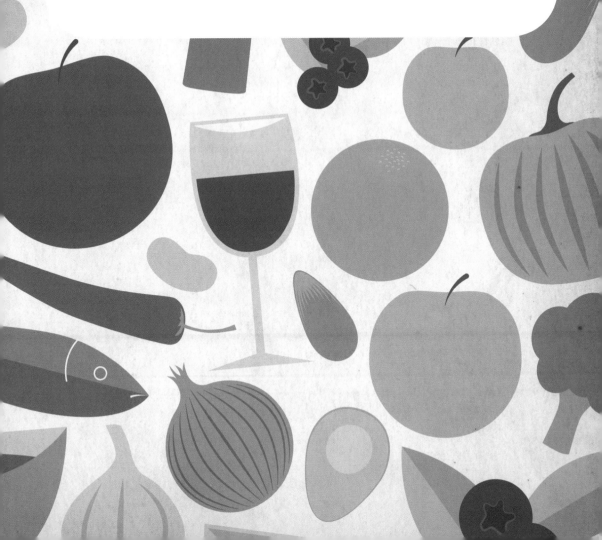

Chapter 11

Mains

There are many types of foods and recipes around the world. It's a lot of fun discovering and trying them out. Hope you enjoy these!

Couscous with Dates, Raisins and Almonds
(Middle Eastern)

This recipe is fruity and nutty – a perfect combination of flavours. It takes about 10 minutes to prepare.

Serves 4

- ❏ 450 ml water
- ❏ 1 tbsp Olivio (or unsalted butter)
- ❏ Grated peel and juice of 1 orange
- ❏ 1 tbsp honey or agave nectar
- ❏ ½ tsp cinnamon
- ❏ ¼ tsp nutmeg
- ❏ ¼ tsp salt
- ❏ 275 g couscous
- ❏ 110 g almonds, sliced
- ❏ 110 g raisins
- ❏ 110 g dates, chopped

1. Mix the water, half the Olivio or butter, orange peel and juice, honey or agave nectar, cinnamon, nutmeg and salt in a medium saucepan and boil.
2. Add the couscous to the boiling mixture. Then remove from the heat and cover for 10 minutes or until all the liquid has been absorbed.
3. In a small frying pan, heat the almonds over a medium heat, stirring continuously until they are toasted. Add the raisins, dates and remaining Olivio or butter. Heat until the butter has melted.
4. Spread the couscous on a serving platter and top with almond and date mixture. Serve on its own or with grilled chicken or fish.

Mains

Baked Curried Fish
(Mtuza Wa Samaki – Kenyan)

A traditional Kenyan recipe for a classic curried stew of fish and onions full of aromatic spices.

Serves 4

- ❏ 900 g sea bass or halibut, bones removed
- ❏ 3 onions, sliced
- ❏ 3 garlic cloves
- ❏ 1 tsp cayenne pepper
- ❏ 1 tbsp curry powder
- ❏ 125 ml white wine vinegar (optional)
- ❏ ½ tsp ground cardamom
- ❏ ½ tsp cumin
- ❏ ½ tsp salt
- ❏ 4 tomatoes
- ❏ 2 tbsp olive oil

1. Preheat the oven to 180°C or Gas Mark 4.
2. Place the fish on a baking tray and add the onions over the fish.
3. In a food processor, mix the garlic, pepper, curry, vinegar, cardamom, cumin and salt until smooth.
4. Add the tomatoes and oil, and blend for just 10 seconds. Avoid blending until smooth.
5. Pour this mixture over the fish. Cover and bake in the oven for 30 minutes or until the fish is cooked. Can be served with wholemeal pitta or with rice.

Mains

Fish with Herbs in Tomato Sauce
(Mauritian)

This is a very rich and delicious sauce, which can be made a bit spicy by adding one chopped serrano chilli. Easy on the lemon with this dish though; use half initially and add the rest if required.

Serves 4

- ❑ 1 kg halibut or sea bass (any white fish is fine), cleaned
- ❑ Salt and pepper to taste
- ❑ 3 tbsp grape seed oil
- ❑ 1 onion, finely chopped
- ❑ 2½ cm ginger, crushed
- ❑ 3 garlic cloves, crushed
- ❑ 10 g fresh thyme, chopped
- ❑ 225 g tomatoes, crushed
- ❑ 2 tbsp tomato paste
- ❑ 125 ml dry sherry
- ❑ 25 g fresh parsley, chopped
- ❑ 25 g fresh coriander, chopped
- ❑ Juice of ½ lemon (optional)

1. Preheat the oven to 150°C or Gas Mark 2.
2. Cut the fish into serving slices and then reassemble to make the whole fish again. Season with salt and pepper to taste. Place the reassembled fish on a baking tray and bake in the oven for 10–15 minutes. Remove from the oven and set aside.
3. Heat the oil in a frying pan. Sauté the onion, ginger, garlic and thyme. Add the crushed tomatoes and tomato paste and mix well. Add salt and pepper to taste. Simmer for 10–15 minutes, then gradually add the sherry.
4. Add half the chopped parsley, coriander and lemon juice. Simmer until the sauce thickens to your preferred consistency.
5. Preheat the oven again to 200°C or Gas Mark 6. Sprinkle the remaining parsley and coriander on the fish in the baking tray.
6. Pour the tomato sauce over the fish evenly then put the fish back in the oven and bake for 10 minutes. Reduce the heat to 150°C and bake for a further 5 minutes. Serve hot with fresh bread or boiled or baked yams.

Spiced Salmon on Lentils
(Moroccan)

A traditional Moroccan recipe for a classic dish of salmon cooked in a spiced tomato-based sauce, served on a bed of lentils. This is a quick and easy recipe that's low in fat and GI.

Serves 4–6

- ❏ 350 g green lentils
- ❏ 1½ litres water
- ❏ ¼ tsp salt
- ❏ ½ tsp freshly ground black pepper
- ❏ 2 tbsp coriander seeds
- ❏ 2 tbsp fennel seeds
- ❏ 2 tbsp cumin seeds
- ❏ 1 tsp cardamom seeds
- ❏ 2 tsp whole cloves
- ❏ 6 tbsp grape seed oil
- ❏ 8 garlic cloves, crushed
- ❏ 2 large shallots, chopped
- ❏ 2 tbsp harissa (Moroccan hot sauce, available in speciality food shops) or any hot sauce
- ❏ 500 g tomatoes, chopped
- ❏ 6 salmon fillets (175 g with skin)
- ❏ 1 tbsp Olivio or unsalted butter

1. Place the lentils in a saucepan and cover with water. Bring to the boil over a high heat. Reduce the heat to low, cover and simmer for 25 minutes, stirring occasionally until the lentils are tender. Season with salt and pepper and set aside, covered.

2. In a frying pan, mix the coriander, fennel, cumin and cardamom seeds with the cloves. Toast the spices over a medium heat for about 3 minutes, stirring until fragrant. Transfer to a plate to cool. Blend the spices in a food processor or with a mortar and pestle.

3. In a saucepan, heat 4 tbsp of grape seed oil over a low heat. Sauté the garlic and shallots for 5 minutes. Add the harissa and 1 tablespoon of the spice mixture and cook, stirring for 3 minutes. Add the tomatoes and juices and simmer over a medium heat for 5 minutes, stirring occasionally. Season with salt and pepper to taste.

4. Preheat the oven to 200°C or Gas Mark 6. Season the salmon with salt and pepper and coat with the remaining spice mixture on both sides.

5. Take 2 ovenproof pans and heat 1 tbsp of oil in each. Add 3 salmon fillets to each pan, skin-side down with a piece of butter next to each fillet and sauté for 3 minutes.

6. Transfer the pans to the oven without turning the salmon and bake for about 6 minutes or until the skins are crisp and the fish is cooked through.

7. Reheat the lentils and tomato sauce. Spoon lentils onto the centre of each dinner plate and place the salmon fillets on top of the lentils. Spoon tomato sauce around the lentils and serve.

Mains

Melon Soup
(Egusi – Nigerian)

There are many variations of making melon soup. It is usually served with ground rice or yams but it can also be served with rice. This recipe can be made with fish as well as meat.

Serves 4

❏ 300 ml water
❏ ½ tsp salt
❏ 1 onion, chopped
❏ 8 chicken pieces
❏ 1 tbsp ground crayfish
❏ 2 tbsp palm oil
❏ 200 g spinach, chopped
❏ 125 g ground melon seeds (egusi)

1. In a saucepan, add the water, salt, onion and chicken, and bring to the boil for 10 minutes.
2. Add the ground crayfish and palm oil and simmer for 10 minutes.
3. Sprinkle over the ground melon seeds and simmer on a low heat for 10–15 minutes, stirring just once.
4. Add the spinach and cook for an additional 5 minutes or until it has just wilted.
5. If you are using fish, add this last and cook for 10 minutes or until the fish is cooked through.

Chicken Tagine with Honey and Apricots (Moroccan)

This recipe is traditionally slow-cooked in a funnel-shaped earthenware tagine. It can be enjoyed with couscous or on its own.

Serves 2–4

- ❑ 2 large onions, chopped
- ❑ 1 whole chicken, cut into small pieces
- ❑ 1 tsp black pepper
- ❑ ½ tsp turmeric
- ❑ 1 cinnamon stick (use 2 sticks if you want a stronger cinnamon aroma and flavour)
- ❑ 450 ml water
- ❑ 450 g dried apricots
- ❑ 2 tsp ground cinnamon
- ❑ 3 tbsp honey or agave nectar
- ❑ 4 tbsp grape seed oil
- ❑ 50 g almonds, peeled
- ❑ 1 tbsp sesame seeds

1. Sauté the onions in a large saucepan until soft.
2. Add the chicken, salt, pepper, turmeric, cinnamon stick and water and bring to the boil. Reduce the heat and simmer for 20 minutes or until the chicken is cooked. Add more water if necessary. Remove the chicken.
3. Add the apricots to the saucepan and simmer for 10 minutes. Add the ground cinnamon and honey or agave. Stir and simmer until the sauce has slightly thickened. Add more honey if necessary.
4. Sauté the almonds in oil for 2 minutes. Drain the oil from the pan, add the sesame seeds and toast.
5. Return the chicken to the saucepan to reheat.
6. To serve, place the chicken on plates. Pour over the sauce and top with almonds and sesame seeds.

Mains

Peanut Sauce with King Prawns and Fragrant Rice (Nigerian)

Serves 2–4

- ❑ 250 g jasmine rice (or any other fragrant rice)
- ❑ 2 red bell peppers, seeds removed
- ❑ 2 red fresh chilli peppers
- ❑ 1 onion, chopped
- ❑ 2½ cm ginger, crushed
- ❑ 1 garlic clove
- ❑ 10 ml water
- ❑ 200 g large king prawns
- ❑ 1 tbsp unsalted peanuts, roasted
- ❑ 10 g fresh thyme, chopped
- ❑ 15 g fresh coriander, chopped
- ❑ 1 chicken stock cube
- ❑ ½ tsp salt
- ❑ ½ tsp black pepper
- ❑ 1 tsp curry powder

1. Boil the rice using the cooking instructions on the packet.
2. In a food processor, blend the red peppers, chilli, onion, ginger, garlic and water until smooth.
3. Pour the mixture into a saucepan and simmer on a low heat for 15–20 minutes. Then add the prawns.
4. Blend the peanuts and herbs in a food processor. Add to the sauce and mix well.
5. Add the chicken stock cube, salt, pepper and the curry powder. Mix and cook for 10 minutes.
6. Spoon the rice onto a plate, top with peanut sauce and serve.

Mains

Chilli Crab with Spinach
(Singaporean)

This recipe is one of Singapore's national dishes. If you enjoy shellfish, you're going to love this crab recipe made with rich-tasting tomato and chilli sauce.

Serves 2–4

- ❏ 1 tbsp ketchup
- ❏ 125 ml water
- ❏ 1 tbsp soy sauce
- ❏ 1 tbsp tomato paste
- ❏ 1 tsp corn flour
- ❏ 1 tbsp sesame oil
- ❏ 2 shallots, chopped
- ❏ 2 garlic cloves, crushed
- ❏ 2½ cm ginger, crushed
- ❏ 1 tbsp red chilli, crushed
- ❏ 200 g baby spinach
- ❏ 450 g crabmeat

1. In a medium bowl, mix the ketchup, water, soy sauce, tomato paste and corn flour.
2. Heat the oil in a saucepan and sauté the shallots for 5 minutes.
3. Add the garlic, ginger and chilli and cook for 1 minute. Add the spinach and cook until just wilted, which takes about 2 minutes.
4. Stir in the sauce and the crabmeat and simmer over a medium heat, stirring occasionally for 5 minutes. Serve with rice.

Mains

Wasabi Salmon Burgers
(Japanese)

Try cooking these over a barbecue. Add some breadcrumbs to add hold. Perfect for a summer's day with any kind of salad.

Serves 2–4

- ❏ 2 tbsp soy sauce
- ❏ 1 tsp wasabi powder (use more if required)
- ❏ ½ tsp honey
- ❏ 450 g salmon fillet, skinned
- ❏ 2 spring onions, chopped
- ❏ 1 egg, lightly beaten
- ❏ 2½ cm ginger, minced
- ❏ 1 tsp sesame oil
- ❏ 4 tbsp grape seed oil

1. Mix the soy sauce, wasabi powder and honey in a small bowl until smooth. Set aside.
2. Chop the salmon with a large knife into 5 mm pieces and transfer to a bowl. Add the spring onions, egg, ginger and sesame oil. Mix thoroughly.
3. Form the mixture into 4 burgers. The mixture will be moist and loose, but it holds together when the first side is cooked.
4. Heat the grape seed oil in a non-stick frying pan over a medium heat. Add the burgers and cook for 5 minutes. Turn and continue to cook until they are firm and fragrant, which takes about 5 minutes.
5. Spoon wasabi sauce evenly over the burgers and cook for a further 30 seconds.

Summer Couscous (Israeli)

Serve hot or cold, with grilled fish or chicken.

Serves 4

- ❑ 225 g couscous
- ❑ 300 ml boiling water
- ❑ 2 carrots, finely chopped
- ❑ 2 celery stalks, finely chopped
- ❑ 1 green pepper, chopped
- ❑ 4 spring onions, chopped
- ❑ 4 sprigs parsley, chopped
- ❑ 50 g raisins
- ❑ 4 tbsp olive oil
- ❑ Juice of ½ lemon
- ❑ 1 garlic clove, crushed
- ❑ ½ tsp salt
- ❑ Black pepper

1. Place the couscous in a medium bowl and add the boiling water. Cover and let stand for about 20 minutes or until the water has been absorbed and the couscous has cooled slightly.
2. Add the finely chopped vegetables, herbs and raisins.
3. In a small bowl, mix the oil, lemon juice, garlic, salt and pepper. Add the mixture to the salad and toss to blend.

Ginger Fried Rice

I tend to vary the type of rice I use when making this recipe. You can try this with Thai, Jasmine or any other fragrant rice. Add some more vegetables such as sweet corn if preferred.

Serves 4–6

- ❑ 3 tsp sesame oil
- ❑ 2 eggs, beaten
- ❑ 6 spring onions, chopped
- ❑ 2½ cm ginger, minced
- ❑ 500 g long-grain brown rice, cooked
- ❑ 150 g frozen peas
- ❑ 100 g mung bean sprouts
- ❑ 2 tbsp oyster sauce

1. Heat 1 tsp of sesame oil in a wok over a medium heat. Add the eggs and scramble. Transfer to a plate and set aside.
2. Pour the remaining oil into the wok. Add the spring onions and ginger and stir fry for about 2 minutes until fragrant. Add the rice and peas and stir fry for about 4 minutes until hot and beginning to stick to the wok.
3. Add the bean sprouts, oyster sauce and the eggs. Stir fry, breaking up the eggs for about 2 minutes. Serve immediately.

Mains

135

Bengali Fish

A Bengali meal without fish is apparently incomplete. Fish is prepared in the most nutritious and delicious way to complement any Bengali meal. Salt and turmeric are the simplest marinade for fish in Bengali cooking.

Serves 4

- ❑ 1 kg cod fillets
- ❑ 1 tsp turmeric
- ❑ 6 tbsp mustard oil or grape seed oil
- ❑ 1 tsp salt
- ❑ 4 fresh green chillies, chopped
- ❑ 2½ cm ginger, crushed
- ❑ 2 garlic cloves, crushed
- ❑ 2 onions, chopped
- ❑ 2 tomatoes, chopped
- ❑ 425 ml water
- ❑ 15 g fresh coriander, chopped

1. Preheat the oven to 180°C or Gas Mark 4.
2. Cut the cod into bite-sized pieces.
3. In a small bowl, mix the turmeric, half the oil and salt together. Pour over the fish. Place on a baking tray and bake for 10 minutes. Remove and set aside.
4. In a food processor, blend the green chilli, ginger, garlic, onions, tomatoes and remaining oil into a paste. Pour into a saucepan and simmer for 10 minutes. Remove from the heat and gently place the fish in the sauce without breaking up the fish.
5. Return the saucepan to a medium heat. Add the water and cook for 15–20 minutes.
6. Garnish with coriander and serve.

Lamb with Potatoes
(Delhi-style)

Serves 4–6

- ❑ 2 tbsp grape seed oil
- ❑ 2 onions, chopped
- ❑ 5 garlic cloves
- ❑ 400 g lamb, diced
- ❑ 400 g tomatoes
- ❑ 1 tbsp cumin
- ❑ 1 tsp coriander
- ❑ ½ tsp turmeric
- ❑ ¼ tsp cayenne pepper
- ❑ 3 tsp salt
- ❑ 400 g potatoes, diced
- ❑ 200 g red lentils
- ❑ 700 ml water

1. Heat the oil in a saucepan and sauté the onion, garlic and lamb for 15 minutes.
2. Add the tomatoes, cumin, coriander, turmeric, pepper and salt. Cook on a high heat for 10–15 minutes.
3. Add the potatoes, lentils and water. Simmer on a low heat for 1 hour and 10 minutes. Serve when cooked.

Chicken Kadai
(Indian)

This is one of my favourites because of the mixture of spices and chilli. Kadai is an Indian cooking pot that looks like a wok, a handle on each side. Serve this with naan bread, chappati, or perhaps with basmati rice.

Serves 4

- ❑ 2 tbsp grape seed oil
- ❑ 1 onion, chopped
- ❑ 2 garlic cloves, chopped
- ❑ 2½ cm ginger, minced
- ❑ 450 g skinless chicken breast, diced
- ❑ 3 tomatoes, peeled and chopped
- ❑ 1 tsp turmeric
- ❑ 2 tsp garam masala
- ❑ ½ tsp chilli powder (or to your taste)
- ❑ Juice of ½ lemon
- ❑ 1 tsp salt
- ❑ 2 tsp coriander to garnish

1. Sauté the onion, garlic and ginger in oil for 10 minutes.
2. Add the chicken, tomatoes, spices, lemon juice and salt. Mix until the chicken is thoroughly coated and sauté for 5 minutes. Cover and simmer over a low heat for 45 minutes.
3. Garnish with coriander and serve.

Curried Lentils with Sweet Potatoes and Spinach

This is a comforting and healthy meal, full of flavour and spices but not fiery hot. Add more curry powder if you like your food spicier.

Serves 4

- ❑ 1 tbsp olive oil
- ❑ 1 onion, chopped
- ❑ 2 garlic cloves, crushed
- ❑ 1 tbsp curry powder
- ❑ 2½ cm ginger, minced
- ❑ 1 tsp ground cumin
- ❑ 200 g dried lentils, rinsed
- ❑ 600 ml vegetable or chicken stock
- ❑ 1 sweet potato, peeled and cut into 5 mm cubes
- ❑ 100 g baby spinach
- ❑ Salt and pepper to taste
- ❑ 225 ml plain yoghurt (optional)
- ❑ 50 g almonds, chopped

1. Heat the oil in a medium saucepan. Add the onion and garlic and sauté for 5 minutes.
2. Stir in the curry powder, ginger and cumin and cook for 1 minute. Add the lentils and stock and bring to the boil. Reduce the heat and simmer, covered, for 10 minutes.
3. Add the sweet potato, cover and cook for 10 minutes until soft.
4. Stir in the spinach and cook for 1 minute until the spinach is just wilted. Add salt and pepper to taste.
5. Transfer to bowls and top each with 1 tbsp of yoghurt and 1 tbsp of chopped almonds. Serve hot.

Tofu with Tomatoes and Coriander

A nutritious recipe especially for vegetarians and vegans. Tofu is an excellent source of protein for vegetarians and vegans and is also rich in calcium and iron.

Serves 4

- ❑ 1 tbsp grape seed oil
- ❑ 6 spring onions, chopped
- ❑ 2 garlic cloves, crushed
- ❑ 3 tomatoes, deseeded and cut into 2½ cm squares
- ❑ 450 g fresh extra firm tofu, drained and cut into 2½ cm squares
- ❑ 1 tsp salt (optional)
- ❑ ½ tsp honey or agave nectar
- ❑ 1 tsp soy sauce
- ❑ ¼ tsp ground coriander
- ❑ ½ tsp black pepper

1. Heat the oil in a wok or saucepan. Stir fry the spring onions and garlic for 2 minutes.
2. Add the tomatoes and stir fry for 1 minute.
3. Add the tofu, salt, honey or agave, soy sauce and coriander. Stir to blend in and cook for 30 seconds.
4. Season with black pepper and serve hot.

Mains

Spicy Salmon Fillets in Tomato and Garlic Sauce

Serves 2–4

- ❏ 2 tsp olive oil
- ❏ 1 onion, coarsely chopped
- ❏ 2 garlic cloves, chopped
- ❏ 1 red bell pepper, chopped
- ❏ 2 tomatoes, coarsely chopped
- ❏ 15 g fresh coriander, chopped
- ❏ 1 can tomatoes, diced
- ❏ 2 tbsp paprika
- ❏ 1 tbsp ground cumin
- ❏ 2 tsp salt
- ❏ 2 tbsp cayenne pepper
- ❏ 1 tsp ground black pepper
- ❏ 125 ml water
- ❏ 450 g salmon fillets, cut into 4 individual slices
- ❏ Juice of ½ lemon

1. Preheat the oven to 180°C or Gas Mark 4.
2. Heat the oil in an ovenproof frying pan and sauté the onion and garlic for 5 minutes.
3. Add the red pepper, chopped fresh tomatoes and coriander. Sauté until tender.
4. In a medium bowl, mix the canned diced tomatoes, 1 tbsp paprika, cumin, salt, 1 tbsp cayenne pepper, ground black pepper and water together thoroughly. Add half the mixture to the pan and cook for 10 minutes.
5. Sprinkle 1 tbsp paprika and 1 tbsp cayenne onto the salmon and rub in. Add the salmon to the sauce and cook for 10 minutes.
6. Pour the remaining tomato mixture over the salmon and continue to cook for another 10 minutes.
7. Add the lemon juice, cover and cook for 5 minutes or until salmon is cooked through.
8. Remove the cover and place the pan in the oven. Broil for 7 minutes and then serve.

Mains

140

Saffron, Courgettes, Peppers and Herb Couscous

Serves 4

- ❑ 300 ml chicken stock
- ❑ 1 tsp salt
- ❑ ½ tsp fresh ground black pepper
- ❑ ¼ tsp ground cumin
- ❑ ½ tsp saffron threads
- ❑ 1 tbsp olive oil
- ❑ 1 tbsp Olivio (or unsalted butter)
- ❑ 2 courgettes, diced
- ❑ 1 onion, chopped
- ❑ 1 red bell pepper, chopped
- ❑ 1 green bell pepper, chopped
- ❑ 250 g couscous
- ❑ 25 g fresh basil, chopped
- ❑ 25 g fresh parsley, chopped

1. Boil the chicken stock in a saucepan and then turn off the heat.
2. Add the salt, pepper, cumin and saffron threads and allow to steep for at least 15 minutes.
3. Heat the olive oil and butter in a saucepan. Add the courgettes, onion, red and green peppers, and cook for 5 minutes or until lightly browned.
4. Bring the stock back to the boil.
5. Place the couscous in a large bowl, add the courgettes and peppers and pour into the hot chicken stock. Cover the bowl tightly with a cover or cling film and leave to stand for 15 minutes.
6. Add the basil and parsley. Using a fork, toss the couscous and herbs. Serve warm.

Mains

Mussels in Tomato and Curry Leaf Sauce (South African)

Serves 4

- ❏ 1 tbsp grape seed oil
- ❏ 2½ cm ginger, chopped
- ❏ 2 garlic cloves, crushed
- ❏ 1 sprig fresh curry leaves
- ❏ 1 can plum tomatoes
- ❏ ½ tsp chilli powder
- ❏ ½ tsp turmeric
- ❏ ½ tsp tamarind paste
- ❏ 200 ml water
- ❏ ½ tsp cumin seeds
- ❏ ½ tsp salt
- ❏ ½ tsp honey or agave nectar
- ❏ 2 kg fresh mussels
- ❏ 1 sprig fresh mint, finely chopped
- ❏ 10 g bean sprouts
- ❏ 1 red chilli, seeds removed, chopped
- ❏ 1 sprig fresh coriander, finely chopped

1. Heat the oil in a large saucepan and sauté the ginger and garlic.
2. Add the curry leaves, tomatoes, chilli powder, turmeric and tamarind. Cook for 2 minutes.
3. Pour in the water and simmer for 10 minutes.
4. Crush the cumin seeds and add to the sauce.
5. Strain the sauce through a sieve. Add the salt and honey or agave.
6. Put the mussels in the sauce and simmer for 3 minutes until they open. Discard any that haven't opened.
7. Place in bowls. Garnish with mint, bean sprouts, red chillies and coriander and serve.

Mains

Halibut with Mediterranean Salsa

You can substitute halibut with any other type of white fish.

Serves 2–4

- ❑ 4 halibut fillets
- ❑ 2 tbsp water
- ❑ ½ tsp chilli powder
- ❑ 1 tsp dried thyme
- ❑ 1 tsp freshly grated lemon zest
- ❑ 1 tomato, deseeded and chopped
- ❑ 1 (60g) can kalamata olives or ripe olives, drained and sliced
- ❑ 15 g fresh parsley, chopped
- ❑ Juice of ½ lemon
- ❑ 1 tbsp capers, drained (optional)
- ❑ 2 tsp extra virgin olive oil
- ❑ 1 tsp dried oregano

1. Preheat the oven to 160°C or Gas Mark 3.
2. Coat a baking dish with cooking oil spray and arrange the fish in a single layer.
3. Pour the water over the fish and sprinkle with chilli powder, thyme and lemon zest. Cover the dish with foil and bake for 15 minutes.
4. In a small bowl, mix the tomato, olives, parsley, lemon juice, capers, oil and oregano thoroughly. Place the fish on a serving platter, top with the salsa and serve.

Mains

Mediterranean Rice and Beans

You can use different types of beans and include vegetables, such as peas, if desired.

Serves 4

- ❑ 2 tbsp olive oil
- ❑ 1 onion, finely chopped
- ❑ 1 garlic clove, crushed
- ❑ 225 g basmati rice, uncooked and washed
- ❑ 2 tsp ground cumin
- ❑ 2 tsp ground coriander
- ❑ 1 tsp turmeric
- ❑ 1 tsp cayenne pepper
- ❑ 1 litre vegetable stock
- ❑ 675 g minced lamb
- ❑ 1 (400g) can chickpeas, drained and rinsed
- ❑ 1 (400g) can black beans, drained and rinsed
- ❑ Juice of 1 lemon
- ❑ 30 g fresh coriander, chopped
- ❑ 15 g fresh parsley, chopped
- ❑ 4 tbsp pine nuts
- ❑ ½ tsp salt
- ❑ ½ tsp ground black pepper

1. Heat 1 tbsp of the olive oil in a medium saucepan. Sauté the onion and garlic for 5 minutes.
2. Add the rice, cumin, coriander, turmeric and cayenne pepper. Cook, stirring constantly for 7 minutes.
3. Add the vegetable stock and bring to the boil. Reduce the heat, cover and simmer for 20 minutes.
4. Sauté the lamb in the remaining olive oil in a saucepan over a medium heat until it is evenly browned.
5. Mix the lamb, chickpeas, black beans, lemon juice, coriander, parsley and pine nuts with the cooked rice. Add salt and pepper to taste. Serve.

Mains

Spicy Mackerel
(Indian)

This recipe gives a spicy zing to the fish and is ideal served with new potatoes and salad. It can be cooked on a barbecue in foil packets rather than in the oven if desired.

Serves 4–6

- ❑ 8 mackerel fillets
- ❑ ½ tsp salt
- ❑ Juice of ½ lime
- ❑ 1 tbsp grapeseed oil
- ❑ 2 carrots, grated
- ❑ ½ tsp ground coriander
- ❑ ½ tsp ground cumin
- ❑ ½ tsp aniseed
- ❑ 1 tsp chilli powder

1. Preheat the oven to 180°C or Gas Mark 4. Line an oven tray with foil and grease the foil. Put the fillets on the tray skin-side down.
2. Rub in the salt and pour over the lime juice. Brush with half the oil and bake for about 5 minutes.
3. Mix the remaining oil, carrots, coriander, cumin, aniseed and chilli. Sprinkle the mixture over the fish and grill for 2 minutes.

Chicken in Spicy Tomato and Herb Sauce
(Indian)

Serves 4

- ❑ 4 chicken breasts, cut in half
- ❑ 1 tbsp salt
- ❑ Juice of ½ lemon
- ❑ 5 garlic cloves, roughly chopped
- ❑ 2½ cm ginger, roughly chopped
- ❑ 2 onions, chopped
- ❑ 4 tbsp grapeseed oil
- ❑ 1 cinnamon stick, halved
- ❑ 4 green cardamom pods, bruised
- ❑ 4 cloves
- ❑ 1 tsp chilli powder
- ❑ ½ tsp turmeric
- ❑ 1 tbsp ground coriander
- ❑ 250g can chopped tomatoes
- ❑ 1 tbsp black peppercorns, coarsely crushed
- ❑ 240 ml warm water

1. Rub the lemon juice and salt into the chicken and set aside.
2. In a food processor, blend the garlic, ginger and onions until smooth.
3. Heat the oil in a large saucepan. Add the cinnamon, cardamom and cloves. Let the spices sizzle gently until the cardamom pods plump up.
4. Add the blended ingredients and stir fry over a medium heat for 5–6 minutes. Reduce the heat and continue stir frying for a further 4 minutes.
5. Add the chilli powder, turmeric, coriander and tomatoes. Cook over a medium heat for 5–6 minutes stirring regularly.
6. Add the black pepper and chicken. Cook over a high heat for about 5 minutes.
7. Pour in the water and bring to the boil. Then reduce the heat, cover and simmer for 25 minutes.
8. Remove the lid and cook for a further 6–8 minutes, until the sauce has reduced to a thick paste. Serve with basmati rice.

Portuguese Rice and Sausage

Portuguese cuisine is characterized by rich, filling and full-flavoured dishes and is closely related to Mediterranean cuisine. I prefer to use Portuguese sausages but if you can't get those, any sausage is fine. I sometimes like to include mixed vegetables such as peas, sweetcorn, carrots, etc.

Serves 4–6

- ❑ 300 g basmati rice
- ❑ 8 Portuguese sausages, cut into thick slices
- ❑ 4 tbsp grape seed oil
- ❑ 1 cinnamon stick
- ❑ 6 green cardamom pods, bruised
- ❑ 6 cloves
- ❑ 1 onion, halved and sliced
- ❑ 3 garlic cloves, crushed
- ❑ 1 tsp chilli powder
- ❑ ½ tsp turmeric
- ❑ 1 green chilli, deseeded and chopped
- ❑ ½ tsp salt
- ❑ 500 ml warm water

1. Wash the rice several times in cold water until clear, then leave to soak in fresh water for 15 minutes.
2. Grill the sausages until browned and cooked through.
3. Heat the oil in a saucepan over a low heat. Add the cinnamon, cardamom and cloves, and let them sizzle until the cardamom pods are plumped up.
4. Add the onion and cook for about 8 minutes until browned. Add the garlic, chilli powder, turmeric and green chilli. Cook for 2–3 minutes.
5. Drain the rice and add it to the saucepan. Stir over a medium heat for 2 minutes then add the salt and pour in the water. Bring to the boil over a high heat.
6. Reduce the heat to medium and cook uncovered for 10–15 minutes until the water has been absorbed. Reduce the heat further to low, mix in the sausages, cover and cook for 6 minutes.
7. Turn the heat off and leave to stand for about 10 minutes before serving.

Mains

Split Peas with Mango Salsa

Split peas are full of potassium, protein and fibre. Combined with all the spices, this recipe creates a nutritious and filling meal.

Serves 4

- ❑ 560 ml water
- ❑ 225 g yellow split peas, rinsed and drained
- ❑ 1 mango, peeled and cubed
- ❑ 110 ml salsa
- ❑ 100 g can pineapple chunks, chopped coarsely
- ❑ 10 g coriander, chopped
- ❑ 2 tsp white wine vinegar
- ❑ Juice of ½ lime
- ❑ ½ tsp ground cumin
- ❑ 2 tbsp olive oil
- ❑ 5 spring onions, chopped
- ❑ ½ tsp powdered ginger
- ❑ ½ tsp ground allspice
- ❑ ¼ tsp ground cardamom
- ❑ Juice of ½ orange
- ❑ 4 tbsp vegetable stock
- ❑ ½ tsp honey or agave nectar
- ❑ 200 g kale, washed and chopped

1. Put the split peas and water in a medium saucepan and bring to the boil over a medium heat. Reduce the heat to low, cover and simmer for 30 minutes or until tender. Drain and set aside.
2. In a medium bowl, mix the mango, salsa, pineapple, coriander, vinegar, lime juice and cumin together. Set aside.
3. Heat 1 tbsp of the oil in a large non-stick frying pan. Add the spring onions and sauté, stirring for 3 minutes.
4. Add the ginger, allspice and cardamom and cook for a minute.
5. Stir in the orange juice, stock and honey or agave nectar. Add the split peas and cook, stirring frequently for 10–15 minutes or until the mixture thickens.
6. In another saucepan, heat the remaining oil, add the kale and cook, stirring constantly for 4–5 minutes or until the kale is just wilted.
7. Place the kale on a serving platter, top with the split peas mixture, then with the mango mixture and serve.

Vegetable Casserole

Good food does not have to be complicated or time-consuming. Use everyday vegetables from the refrigerator for a warming and heart-healthy meal.

••

Serves 4

- ❑ Peel and juice of 1 orange
- ❑ 2 tsp corn flour
- ❑ 6 sweet potatoes, cut into cubes
- ❑ 2 onions, cut into 6 wedges
- ❑ 2 leeks, thickly sliced
- ❑ 2 carrots, peeled and sliced into 1 cm thick rounds
- ❑ 150 g pitted prunes, halved
- ❑ 225g can unsweetened pineapple chunks
- ❑ 1 cm ginger, chopped
- ❑ 1 tsp ground cinnamon
- ❑ 4 tbsp toasted almonds, chopped

1. Preheat the oven to 190°C or Gas Mark 5. Coat a baking dish with non-stick spray.
2. In a large bowl, mix the orange juice and corn flour until smooth.
3. Add the orange peel, sweet potatoes, onions, leeks, carrots, prunes, pineapple chunks with juice, ginger and cinnamon. Mix well to blend, pour into the baking dish and cover with foil.
4. Bake in the oven for 45 minutes.
5. Remove the foil and sprinkle with almonds. Bake for another 15 minutes and serve.

Greek Stuffed Tomatoes

Add more herbs and spices to create your own unique version. This can be served as a starter as well.

••

Serves 3–6

- ❑ 2 tbsp olive oil
- ❑ 1 onion, chopped
- ❑ 100 g spinach, chopped
- ❑ Handful of parsley, chopped
- ❑ 2 tsp dried basil
- ❑ ½ tsp crushed chilli (optional)
- ❑ 50 g breadcrumbs
- ❑ 225 g feta cheese, crumbled
- ❑ ½ tsp salt
- ❑ ½ tsp black pepper
- ❑ 6 large tomatoes, firm and insides scooped out

1. Preheat the oven to 180°C or Gas Mark 4.
2. Heat the oil in a saucepan over a medium heat and sauté the onion for 5 minutes. Add the spinach and cook for 2 minutes.
3. In a bowl, mix the onion, spinach, parsley, basil, crushed chilli, breadcrumbs, cheese, salt and pepper together.
4. Stuff the mixture into the tomatoes and bake for 15 minutes. Serve.

Seafood Stew

A rustic yet sophisticated seafood stew that will be a winner with both family and dinner party guests.

Serves 4

- ❑ 4 tbsp olive oil
- ❑ 1 onion, chopped
- ❑ 3 celery stalks, chopped
- ❑ 1 green bell pepper, chopped
- ❑ 1 red bell pepper, chopped
- ❑ 5 garlic cloves, crushed
- ❑ ½ tsp red pepper, crushed
- ❑ 2 tsp dried oregano
- ❑ 1 tsp dried marjoram
- ❑ 3 tbsp fresh basil, chopped
- ❑ 450 ml bottled clam juice
- ❑ 2 cans (425 g) chopped tomatoes
- ❑ 140 ml red wine
- ❑ 450 g white fish, cut into cubes (halibut, haddock or cod)
- ❑ 450g king prawns, shelled and de-veined
- ❑ 450 g scallops (washed and cut in half) or mussels (pre-cooked, removed from shells and cut in half)
- ❑ Juice of ½ lemon
- ❑ ½ tsp salt and coarsely ground black pepper
- ❑ Grated parmesan or romano cheese to garnish

1. Heat the oil in a medium saucepan over a medium heat. Add the onion and sauté for 5 minutes.
2. Add the celery and peppers and sauté for 2 minutes.
3. Stir in the garlic, crushed pepper, oregano, marjoram and basil. Lower the heat and cook for 2 minutes.
4. Add the clam juice, tomatoes and wine. Cover and simmer for 15 minutes.
5. Add the fish, prawns, scallops or mussels. Cook for 4–5 minutes or until the seafood is just cooked.
6. Stir in the lemon juice and season with salt and pepper to taste. Garnish with grated parmesan or romano.

Russo's Ratatouille
(South African)

Serves 4

- ❑ 4 tbsp olive oil
- ❑ 1 onion, chopped
- ❑ 5 garlic cloves, crushed
- ❑ 1 bay leaf
- ❑ 1 aubergine, washed and cubed
- ❑ 1 tsp salt
- ❑ 15 g fresh basil, chopped
- ❑ 2 tsp dried oregano
- ❑ 1 tsp rosemary
- ❑ 2 courgettes, washed and cubed
- ❑ 2 yellow squash, washed and cubed
- ❑ 1 red bell pepper, deseeded and chopped
- ❑ 1 green bell pepper, deseeded and chopped
- ❑ 3 tomatoes, chopped
- ❑ 125 ml dry red wine
- ❑ 225 g mushrooms, sliced
- ❑ 15 g fresh parsley, chopped
- ❑ 2 tbsp parmesan cheese, grated (optional)

1. Heat the olive oil in a saucepan. Add the onion, garlic and bay leaf, and sauté for 5 minutes.
2. Add the aubergine, salt, basil, oregano and rosemary. Cover and cook over a medium heat for 10 minutes, stirring occasionally.
3. Add the courgettes, yellow squash, peppers, tomatoes and wine. Cover and simmer over a low heat for 10 minutes.
4. Mix in the mushrooms and parsley. Simmer for 5 minutes or until the vegetables are tender.
5. Remove the bay leaf. Serve on a plate and garnish with parmesan.

Mains

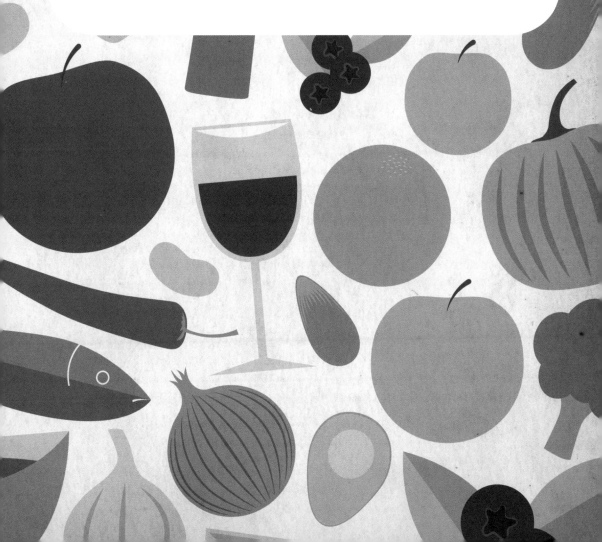

Chapter 12

Desserts

A few of these desserts include fruit and some also include digestive aids such as fennel and ginger. Enjoy!

Creamy Dark Chocolate and Almond Mousse

This recipe is courtesy of Kristen Suzanne of kristenraw.com. It's a fabulous dessert, packed full of nutrients, vitamins and minerals. You can use any other flavour of extract – try orange, it's fantastic!

Serves 4

- ❑ 75 ml water
- ❑ 1 tsp almond extract
- ❑ 2 tbsp honey or agave nectar
- ❑ 125 g dark chocolate powder (more than 70 percent cocoa)
- ❑ 2 avocados, deseeded and peeled
- ❑ 2 tbsp almonds, crushed
- ❑ 1 sprig mint (garnish)

1. In a food processor, blend the water, almond extract, honey or agave nectar, chocolate and avocados until smooth.
2. Spoon into goblets or ice cream bowls and refrigerate for an hour or until ready to serve.
3. Sprinkle with crushed almonds and garnish with 1 mint leaf per serving.

Coconut Candy
(Nigerian)

This used to be a firm favourite growing up. I remember making coconut candy some days after school at home.

Serves 6–8

- ❑ 4 tbsp honey or agave nectar (or 1 tbsp unrefined brown sugar)
- ❑ 2 coconuts, flesh shredded (or 700 g dried coconut)
- ❑ 2 tbsp water

1. In a saucepan, heat the honey or agave.
2. Mix the coconut and water in a bowl and add to the saucepan. Cook for about 5 minutes, stirring continuously. Remove from the heat and allow to cool a little.
3. Scoop 1 or 2 tablespoons into the palm of your hand and roll into a ball. Place on a platter and repeat using all the mixture. Allow to cool completely and harden.

Baked Bananas

Serves 6–8

- ❏ 4 tbsp fresh orange juice
- ❏ 1 tbsp flour
- ❏ 2 tbsp honey or agave nectar
- ❏ 3 tbsp cinnamon
- ❏ 8 bananas, cut diagonally into 3 pieces
- ❏ 250 ml sour cream
- ❏ 110 g coconut, shredded

1. Preheat the oven to 180°C or Gas Mark 4.
2. In a small bowl, mix the orange juice, flour, honey or agave and half the cinnamon until smooth.
3. Place the bananas in an ovenproof dish and glaze with the syrup.
4. Cover with foil and bake for 10 minutes.
5. Place a piece of banana in each individual compote dish and top with 3 tbsp of sour cream. Dust with cinnamon and sprinkle with 1 tbsp of coconut.

Fruit Salad

Serves 4–6

- ❏ ½ melon, cubed
- ❏ 2 apples, cored and cubed
- ❏ 2 bananas, sliced
- ❏ 5 oranges, peeled, deseeded and chopped
- ❏ Juice of 3 oranges
- ❏ Juice of 1 lemon
- ❏ 1½ tbsp honey or agave nectar
- ❏ 1 tsp vanilla essence
- ❏ 1 tsp cinnamon

Mix all the ingredients in a large bowl. Chill before serving.

Mango and Banana Sundae

Serves 2–4

- ❏ 1 mango, peeled and chopped
- ❏ 2 bananas, peeled and chopped
- ❏ Juice of ½ lemon
- ❏ Juice of 2 oranges
- ❏ Vanilla ice cream

1. In a medium bowl, mix the mango, bananas, lemon juice and orange juice together.
2. Spoon the fruit salad into ice cream bowls, top with a scoop of ice cream and serve.

Watermelon with Fennel Seeds

The best dessert you can have to aid digestion. Fennel seeds often provide quick and effective relief from digestive disorders.

Serves 4–6

- ❏ 1 tbsp fennel seeds
- ❏ 2 tsp salt
- ❏ 1 watermelon, quartered and cut into 2½ cm thick slices
- ❏ 2 limes, cut into wedges

1. Heat a frying pan over a low heat for about 3 minutes until hot. Add the fennel seeds and toast, stirring constantly for 3–4 minutes. Transfer to a plate and allow to cool.
2. In a food processor or using a mortar and pestle, crush the fennel seeds.
3. Mix the seeds with salt and sprinkle over the watermelon. Serve with lime wedges.

Desserts

Green Tea Poached Pears with Cream

Serves 4

- ❑ 850 ml water
- ❑ 1½ tbsp green tea leaves
- ❑ 3 tbsp honey or agave nectar
- ❑ 1 tbsp crystallized ginger, chopped
- ❑ ½ tsp almond extract
- ❑ 4 firm, ripe pears, halved and cored
- ❑ 1 tbsp sliced almonds, toasted
- ❑ 125 ml single cream

1. Bring the water to the boil in a saucepan. Add the green tea leaves and stir. Turn off the heat and cover, allowing to steep for 5 minutes.
2. Pour through a sieve into a bowl to remove the leaves and return to the saucepan.
3. Add the honey or agave, ginger and almond extract, and bring to the boil.
4. Add the pears, cut side up, and poach over a low heat until quite tender when pierced with a fork.
5. Transfer to a bowl and let the pears cool in the liquid. Chill for 30 minutes.
6. Place 2 pear halves in each dessert dish. Pour 2 tbsp of sauce over the pears, top with 2 tbsp of cream and garnish with almonds.

Spiced Dried Fruit Compote

As well as a nutritious dessert ingredient, dried fruit is the perfect snack to eat between meals.

Serves 2–4

- ❑ 225 ml water
- ❑ 1 green teabag
- ❑ 175 g dried apricots, halved
- ❑ 110 g dried figs, halved
- ❑ 110 g dried cherries
- ❑ 1 tbsp honey
- ❑ 1 cm ginger
- ❑ 1 strip lemon rind
- ❑ 1 small cinnamon stick

1. In a medium saucepan, bring the water to the boil and then remove from the heat.
2. Add the teabag and allow to steep for 5 minutes. Remove and discard the bag.
3. Add the apricots, figs, cherries, honey, ginger, lemon rind and cinnamon stick. Bring to the boil.
4. Reduce the heat to low and simmer, stirring occasionally, for 15–20 minutes or until the fruit is tender.
5. Remove and discard the ginger, lemon rind and cinnamon stick. Serve warm or chilled.

Desserts

157

Pears in Red Wine

A very delicious and easy to prepare dessert that can be made the day before.

Serves 4

- ❏ 4 firm pears, washed and peeled, saving the skin
- ❏ 500 ml red wine
- ❏ 2 tbsp agave nectar or unrefined brown sugar
- ❏ 1 cinnamon stick
- ❏ Cream or ice cream (optional)

1. Place the pears and skins in a large saucepan and add the wine, agave or sugar and the cinnamon. Bring to the boil over a medium heat for about 20 minutes, turning the pears over.
2. Remove the pears from the liquid, place in a dish and set aside.
3. Continue cooking the red wine with the skins and cinnamon, slowly reducing the liquid until all the alcohol has evaporated and the liquid consistency is thick.
4. Remove the cinnamon and pear skins from the syrup and cook further for 5 minutes.
5. Add the pears to the syrup and cook for 5 minutes.
6. Turn off the heat and let the pears cool to room temperature.
7. Place in individual dessert bowls and top with syrup. Serve plain or with ice cream or cream.

Desserts

Spiced Oranges

Serves 4–6

- ❑ 4 tbsp honey or agave nectar (or 2 tbsp unrefined brown sugar)
- ❑ 2 cloves
- ❑ 1 cinnamon stick
- ❑ 1 cm ginger, sliced thinly
- ❑ 500 ml carton orange juice (preferably Tropicana or fresh juice)
- ❑ 6 oranges, peeled, pith and pips removed, and sliced thinly
- ❑ Fresh cream to serve
- ❑ Toasted flaked almonds

1. Place all the ingredients in a saucepan except the sliced oranges, cream and flaked almonds. Bring to a boil and simmer on a low heat for 1½ hours, stirring occasionally, or until the mixture thickens like syrup.
2. Mix in the orange slices and transfer to a bowl.
3. Serve in dessert bowls. Top each with 1 tbsp of cream and sprinkle with 1 tbsp of flaked almonds.

Chapter 13

Smoothies, Juices and Shots

Make these using a blender or smoothie maker. I use the Kenwood Smoothie Pro, which I find quite easy to use and clean. I also use the Phillips HR1865 for juicing. It's one of the best juicers I have used and pretty easy to clean.

Smoothies

Cleanse Smoothie

This smoothie is packed full of vitamins and minerals to nourish and cleanse the body. The lemon and lime, which are known for their cleansing properties, contain acid which scours the intestinal tract eliminating toxins and neutralizing harmful bacteria. Celery and cucumber are known for their excellent diuretic properties, which aid in reducing fluid retention and help reduce blood pressure. This juice can also be made using a juicer. Do not juice if you are adding avocado.

- 100g baby spinach, washed
- Juice of 1 lemon
- Juice of 1 lime
- 1 cucumber
- 3 celery sticks
- 1 apple
- 1 cm ginger
- 1 kiwi, peeled (optional)
- ½ avocado (optional)
- ½ tsp honey or agave nectar (optional)

Put all ingredients except the honey or agave in a smoothie maker and blend until smooth. If you are using a juicer, do not include the avocado because avocados cannot be juiced. Add the honey or agave only if the mixture is a bit sour to your taste. Add ice cubes and crush for a more refreshing smoothie.

Peach, Spinach and Mint Smoothie

The addition of mint in this smoothie promotes digestion. Peaches are good for cleansing the intestine, bladder and kidneys.

- 100g spinach, washed (preferably baby spinach)
- 2 peaches, peeled, cored and cubed
- 3 sprigs mint, washed
- 1 apple, peeled, cored and cubed
- Juice of ½ lemon
- ½ cucumber, peeled if not organic
- 1 tsp honey or agave nectar

Place all ingredients in a smoothie maker and blend until smooth. It tastes even better with crushed ice.

Antioxidant Boost

Berries have a high antioxidant effect which aids in destroying free radicals, boosting the immune system and slowing down the signs of ageing.

- 75g blueberries, washed
- 75g raspberries, washed
- 1 banana, peeled and chopped
- 10 strawberries, stems removed and washed
- Juice of 1 orange
- 50 g pomegranate (½ pomegranate with fruit squeezed out)
- ½ tsp honey or agave nectar (optional)

Place all ingredients in a smoothie maker and blend until smooth.

Pineapple Blast

This is a fantastic cold remedy, full of Vitamin C and a great decongestant. Pineapple contains an enzyme called bromeline which helps dissolve excess mucous. I make this as a smoothie as I want to taste everything but it can also be juiced if preferred.

- 1 pineapple, peeled and chopped
- Juice of 1 lemon
- 2½ cm ginger
- 1 tbsp manuka honey

Blend all ingredients in a smoothie maker or juicer.

Super-Charged Cinnamon

Bee pollen has a high concentration of vitamin B complex as well as vitamins A, C, D and E.

- ❑ ½ blender of almond or rice milk
- ❑ 75g berries (blueberries, cherries or raspberries)
- ❑ 1 avocado
- ❑ 1 banana
- ❑ 3 heaped tbsp fresh bee pollen
- ❑ 1 tbsp raw, organic honey
- ❑ 4 tbsp ground sprouted flax powder
- ❑ 1 tsp cinnamon

1. Half fill your blender with the almond or rice milk. Add all the ingredients except for the flax powder and cinnamon. Turn the blender on low until the mixture is smooth.
2. Add the flax powder and cinnamon and blend well on high for 2 minutes until creamy.

Popeye's Power Punch

This smoothie is good for boosting the immune system and vitamin B3 is an excellent aid for brain and nerve function. Alfalfa sprouts are rich in silicon, excellent for the growth of strong and healthy hair.

- ❑ ½ bunch of celery
- ❑ 1 bag of spinach
- ❑ ½ green pepper
- ❑ ½ cucumber
- ❑ 30 g parsley, chopped
- ❑ 1 avocado
- ❑ 1 scoop alfalfa
- ❑ 1 scoop bean sprouts
- ❑ 4 tbsp fresh coriander, chopped
- ❑ 1 small tomato
- ❑ 2 spring onions, chopped (optional)
- ❑ 80 ml water
- ❑ 6 ice cubes

Place all the ingredients in a blender, one by one, and blend until creamy smooth. Add the ice cubes last. Alternatively, you can make this in a saucepan on your hob using a low temperature. Stir constantly as if you are making a soup. Leave out the ice cubes to make a warm smoothie.

Strawberry Sunrise

Serve chilled as a wonderful vitamin-packed breakfast.

- ❑ 10 fresh strawberries
- ❑ 1 banana
- ❑ 4 rings of freshly sliced pineapple
- ❑ 225 ml organic soya plain yoghurt
- ❑ A few ice cubes

Place all ingredients in a blender and blend until creamy smooth. Add the ice cubes and, if necessary, a splash of water to reach the right consistency.

Pumpin-Jumpin-Power

A good breakfast smoothie to energize and boost the immune system. It can also aid in reducing blood pressure and reduce inflammation in the body.

- ❑ 1 large banana
- ❑ 8 tbsp organic oat bran – not porridge oats
- ❑ 1 heaped tbsp sprouted flax powder
- ❑ 225 ml unsweetened soya milk or almond milk
- ❑ 1 heaped tsp of organic honey
- ❑ ¼ tsp cinnamon powder

Place all ingredients in a blender and blend until smooth. Add a splash more milk or water if the consistency is not right for your personal taste.

Fabulous Fig Fest

If you are using dried figs, soak them in water for at least 30 minutes first.

- ❑ 5 dried or fresh figs
- ❑ ½ mango
- ❑ ½ avocado
- ❑ 4 tbsp ground sprouted flax powder
- ❑ ½ pineapple, cut into chunks
- ❑ 225 ml fresh apple juice
- ❑ Ice cubes as needed

Put all ingredients in a blender and blend on high for 3 minutes if you are using dried figs, 2 minutes if you are using fresh figs. Adjust the number of ice cubes to your taste.

Tantalizing Tart

I wouldn't let this one sit around – so only make as much as you are going to drink right away.

- ❑ 2 cucumbers
- ❑ 2 hard Granny Smith's apples
- ❑ 1 head of kale (about 7 leaves) or 1 bag (200 g) of spinach
- ❑ 1 lemon, remove the skin but keep the white pith

Juice everything in a blender or smoothie maker and enjoy!

Juices

Super C for Energy

To boost energy, aid digestion and improve skin care. This juice is high in fibre, vitamins A and C, lycopene, beta-carotene and tryptophan.

- ❑ 4 florets of broccoli
- ❑ 1 red pepper
- ❑ ½ cucumber
- ❑ Juice of 1 lime
- ❑ Handful of parsley

Green Mamba

Good for anaemia, constipation and cleansing the body of toxins. Packed full of vitamins A, C, B and K, it also contains iron and anti-inflammatory properties.

- ❑ ½ bag of spinach
- ❑ 2 celery stalks
- ❑ ½ fennel
- ❑ ½ cucumber
- ❑ Juice of 1 lime
- ❑ 1 cm ginger

166

It's Good for You!

Lowers blood pressure and oxygenates the blood, offers high levels of anti-carcinogens and is a good diuretic. Contains vitamins A, B, C and K, and is rich in iron, sulphur and fibre.

....

- ❑ ½ beetroot
- ❑ ½ bag of spinach
- ❑ 2 carrots

- ❑ ¼ cabbage
- ❑ 2 celery stalks
- ❑ 2 tsp flax oil

The Lion Sleeps Tonight!

Aids digestion, insomnia, scurvy, skin and eye care, and keeps the body alkaline. Rich in vitamins A, B and C.

....

- ❑ 4 stalks of celery
- ❑ ½ cucumber

- ❑ Juice of 1 lime
- ❑ Handful of mint

Heart Smart

Natural diuretic, aids digestion and is good for flatulence. High in vitamins A, C, B and K.

....

- ❑ 1 cm ginger
- ❑ Handful of mint
- ❑ Handful of parsley

- ❑ 4 celery stalks
- ❑ ½ fennel

Sweet Flush

Reduces pain and fever, improves hair, skin and nails, and eases cramps and gout.

....

- ❑ Handful of mint
- ❑ Juice of 1 lime
- ❑ 1 cucumber

- ❑ ½ fennel
- ❑ ½ beetroot (optional)

Mootli for Mucous

Removes stomach mucous, relieves constipation, lowers blood pressure, oxygenates the blood and cleanses the body of toxins.

- ❑ 10 cm mooli (can be found in Japanese shops)
- ❑ ½ bag of mint
- ❑ ½ beetroot
- ❑ 1 carrot
- ❑ 1 cm ginger

Green Gunge

High in iron and anti-inflammatory properties, aids digestion, eases diarrhoea, arthritis and acts as a natural diuretic.

- ❑ ½ bag of spinach
- ❑ ½ fennel
- ❑ ½ cucumber
- ❑ 5 florets of broccoli
- ❑ 2 celery stalks
- ❑ Handful of parsley
- ❑ 1 cm ginger

Shots

Make these using a juicer.

Tula-Tula

This will make you sleep like a baby.

- ❏ 1 celery stalk
- ❏ Juice of ½ lime
- ❏ 1 tsp honey

Ding-Dong

Kick starts the entire body.

- ❏ 1 cm ginger
- ❏ ½ tsp cinnamon
- ❏ ½ tsp turmeric
- ❏ 1 lemon or lime, juice and rinds

Oh Gracious Gut

Gets rid of tummy mucous.

- ❏ 5 cm mooli
- ❏ Juice of ½ lime
- ❏ Handful of mint
- ❏ 5 cm cucumber

Depressurization Sensation

Instantly lowers blood pressure.

- ❏ ½ beetroot
- ❏ Juice of ½ lemon
- ❏ 2½ cm ginger

Bibliography

Almonds

Sofi F, Cesari F, Abbate R, Gensini GF and Casini A (2008) 'Adherence to Mediterranean diet and health status: meta-analysis'. *BMJ* (Clinical research ed.). 337: a1344.

Apples

Puel C, Quintin A, Mathey J, Obled C, Davicco MJ, Lebecque P, Kati-Coulibaly S, Horcajada MN and Coxam V (2005) 'Prevention of bone loss by phloridzin, an apple polyphenol, in ovariectomized rats under inflammation conditions'. *Calcified Tissue International.* 77(5): 311–18.

School of Public Health, University of California, Los Angeles (2008) 'Fruits, vegetables, teas may protect smokers from lung cancer'. Press Release, 29 May. www.ph.ucla.edu/pr/newsitem052908.html

Liu RH, Liu J and Chen B (2005) 'Apples prevent mammary tumors in rats'. *Journal of Agricultural and Food Chemistry.* 53(6): 2341–43.

Aubergines

Murray M, Pizzorno J and Pizzorno L (2008) *The Encyclopaedia of Healing Foods.* London: Piatkus Books.

Matsubara K, Kaneyuki T, Miyake T and Mori M (2005) 'Antiangiogenic activity of nasunin, an antioxidant anthocyanin, in eggplant peels'. *Journal of Agricultural and Food Chemistry.* 53(16): 6272–75.

Kwon YI, Apostolidis E and Shetty K (2008) 'In vitro studies of eggplant (Solanum melongena) phenolics as inhibitors of key enzymes relevant for type 2 diabetes and hypertension'. *Bioresource Technology.* 99(8): 2981–88.

Gallop R (2005) *The GI Pocket Guide.* London: Virgin Books.

Avocado

Lu QY, Arteaga JR, Zhang Q, Huerta S, Go VLW and Heber D (2005) 'Inhibition of prostate cancer cell growth by an avocado extract: role of lipid-soluble bioactive substances'. *The Journal of Nutritional Biochemistry*. 16(1): 23–30.

Murray M, Pizzorno J and Pizzorno L (2008) *The Encyclopaedia of Healing Foods*. London: Piatkus Books.

Bananas

American Academy of Neurology (2002) 'Will A Banana A Day Keep A Stroke Away? Low Potassium Intake May Increase Stroke Risk.' ScienceDaily. 13 August. www.sciencedaily.com/releases/2002/08/020813072509.htm

Beans

Bennink M 'Eat beans for good health'. Bean Improvement Cooperative, Michigan State University. www.css.msu.edu/bic/pdf/nutrition.pdf

Cabbage

Fowke JH, Longcope C and Herbert JR (2000) 'Brassica vegetable consumption shifts estrogen metabolism in healthy postmenopausal women'. Cancer Epidemiology, Biomarkers & Prevention. 9: 773. cebp.aacrjournals.org/content/9/8/773.full

Adzersen KH, Jess P, Freivogel KW, Gerhard I and Bastert G (2003) 'Raw and cooked vegetables, fruits, selected micronutrients, and breast cancer risk: A case-control study in Germany'. *Nutrition and Cancer*. 46(2): 131–37.

Cheney G (1949) 'Rapid healing of peptic ulcers in patients receiving fresh cabbage juice'. California Medicine. 70(1): 10–15. www.ncbi.nlm.nih.gov/pmc/articles/PMC1643665/pdf/califmed00295-0012.pdf

Cardamom

Yadav AS and Bhatnagar D (2007) 'Free radical scavenging activity, metal chelation and antioxidant power of some of the Indian spices'. *Biofactors*. 31(3–4): 219–27.

Bhattacharjee S, Rana T and Sengupta (2007) 'An inhibition of lipid per oxidation and enhancement of GST activity by cardamom and cinnamon during chemically induced colon carcinogenesis in Swiss albino mice.' *Asian Pacific Journal of Cancer Prevention.* 8(4): 578–82.

Carrots

Baer HJ, Schnitt SJ, Connolly JL, Byrne C, Cho E, Willett WC and Colditz GA (2003) 'Adolescent Diet and Incidence of Proliferative Benign Breast Disease'. *Cancer Epidemiology, Biomarkers & Prevention.* 12: 1159.

Cinnamon

Schoene NW, Kelly MA, Polansky MM and Anderson RA (2005) 'Water-soluble polymeric polyphenols from cinnamon inhibit proliferation and alter cell cycle distribution patterns of hematologic tumor cell lines'. *Cancer Letters.* 230(1): 134–40.

Scott K (2006) *Medicinal Seasonings: The Healing Power of Spices.* Cape Town: Medspice Press.

Citrus

Enonomos C and Clay WD (1999) 'Nutritional and health benefits of citrus fruits'. *Journal of Food, Nutrition and Agriculture.* 24: 11–18.

Béliveau R and Gingras D (2007) *Foods to Fight Cancer.* London: Dorling Kindersley.

Corn

Dewanto V, Wu X and Liu RH (2002) 'Processed sweet corn has higher antioxidant activity'. *Journal of Agricultural and Food Chemistry. Journal of Agricultural and Food Chemistry.* 50(17): 4959–64.

Courgettes

Edenharder R, Kurz P, John K, et al. (1994) 'In vitro effect of vegetable and fruit juices on the mutagenicity of 2- amino-3-methylimidazo[4,5-f] quinoline, 2-amino-3,4-dimethylimidazo[4,5- f]quinoline and 2-amino-3,8-dimethylimidazo[4,5-f]quinox'. *Food and Chemical Toxicology.* 32(5): 443–59.

Cumin

Martinez-Tome M, Jimenez AM, Ruggieri S, et al. (2001) 'Antioxidant properties of Mediterranean spices compared with common food additives'. *Journal of Food Protection*. 64(9): 1412–19.

Kawther S, Zaher W, Ahmed M and Zerizer SN (2008) 'Observations on the Biological Effects of Black Cumin Seed (Nigella sativa) and Green Tea (Camellia sinensis)'. *Global Veterinaria*. 2(4): 198–204.

Scott K (2006) *Medicinal Seasonings: The Healing Power of Spices*. Cape Town: Medspice Press.

Fenugreek

Basch E, Ulbricht C, Kuo G, Szapary P and Smith M (2003) 'Therapeutic Applications of Fenugreek'. *Alternative Medicine Review*. 8(1): 20–7.

Fish

British Medical Journal 2004; 328 doi: 10.1136/bmj. 328.7430. 0-e (published 1 January 2004).

Flaxseed

Cunnane SC, Hamadeh MJ, Liede AC, Thompson LU, Wolever TM and Jenkins DJ (1995) 'Nutritional attributes of traditional flaxseed in healthy young adults'. *American Journal of Clinical Nutrition*. 61: 62–8. www.ajcn.org/cgi/reprint/61/1/62

Serraino M and Thompson LU (1992) 'Flaxseed supplementation and early markers of colon carcinogenesis'. *Cancer Letters*. 63(2): 159–65.

Garlic

Lazovich, D, Robien K, Cutler, G, Virnig, B and Sweeney, C (2009) 'Quality of life in a prospective cohort of elderly women with and without cancer'. *Cancer. Survivorship Research: Mapping the New Challenges*. 115: S18: 4283–97. http://onlinelibrary.wiley.com/doi/10.1002/cncr.24580/full

Ginger

Rhode J, Fogoros S, Zick S, Wahl H, Griffith KA, Huang J and Liu JR (2007) 'Ginger inhibits cell growth and modulates angiogenic factors in ovarian cancer cells'. BMC Complementary and Alternative Medicine. 7: 44. www.biomedcentral.com/1472-6882/7/44

Béliveau, R and Gingras, D (2007) *Foods to Fight Cancer*. London: Dorling Kindersley.

Goji Berries

Moss R (2004) 'A Friendly Skeptic Looks at Goji Juice'. *CancerDecisions Newsletter*, 21 Nov. www.cancerdecisions.com/112104.html
www.gojijuices.net/gojijuiceresearch.html

Grape Seed Oil

Nakamura Y, Tsuji S and Tonogai Y (2003) 'Analysis of proanthocyanidins in grape seed extracts, health foods and grape seed oils'. *Journal of Health Science*. 49(1): 45–54.

Green Peas

Sultan N, Khan MA and Malik S (2004) 'Effect of folic acid supplementation on homocysteine level in postmenopausal women'. *Human Reproduction*. 19(4): 1031–35.

Paradisi G, Cucinelli F, Mele MC, Barini A, Lanzone A and Caruso A (2004) 'Endothelial function in post-menopausal women: effect of folic acid supplementation'. *Human Reproduction*. 19(4): 1031–35.

Kunkler IH (2006) 'Folic acid and breast cancer'. *Journal of the Royal College of Physicians of Edinburgh*. 36: 35–7. www.rcpe.ac.uk/journal/issue/journal_36_1/H_follic_acid_kunkler.pdf

Kale

British Medical Journal, 2004 May 29: 328 (7451): 1285.43. Sarkar FH, LiY.

Leeks

Ensminger AH, Esminger MKJ, et al. (1986) *Food for Health: A Nutrition Encyclopaedia*. Clovis, CA: Pegus Press.

Manach C, Scalbert A, Morand C, Rémésy C, Jiménez L (2004) 'Polyphenols: food sources and bioavailability'. *American Journal of Clinical Nutrition*. 79(5): 727–47.

Mint

Dr Duke's Phytochemical and Ethnobotanical databases: www.ars-grin.gov/duke/

Miso

Béliveau, R and Gingras, D (2007) *Foods to Fight Cancer*. London: Dorling Kindersley.

Belleme J and Belleme J (2007) *Japanese Foods that Heal*. North Clarendon, VT: Tuttle.

Mushrooms

Stengle M (2005) *The Health Benefits of Medicinal Mushrooms*. Laguna Beach, CA: Basic Health Publications.

Grube BJ, Eng ET, Kao YC, et al. (2001) 'White Button Mushroom Phytochemicals Inhibit Aromatase Activity and Breast Cancer Cell Proliferation'. *Journal of Nutrition*. 131(12): 3288–93.

Pomegranate

Longtin R 'The Pomegranate: Nature's Power Fruit?' (2003) *Journal of the National Cancer Institute*. 95(5): 346–48.

Quinoa

Anderson JW (2004) 'Whole grains and coronary heart disease: the whole kernel of truth'. *American Journal of Clinical Nutrition*. 80(6): 1459–60.

Cade JE, Burley VJ and Greenwood DC (2007) 'Dietary fibre and risk of breast cancer in the UK Women's Cohort Study'. *International Journal of Epidemiology*.

36(2): 431–38.

Wood, R (1988) *The Whole Foods Encyclopedia*. New York, NY: Prentice-Hall Press.

Red Wine

Szmitko PE and Verma S (2005) 'Red Wine and Your Heart'. *Circulation, Journal of the American Heart Association*. 111: e10–e11. www.circ.ahajournals.org/cgi/reprint/111/2/e10

Saffron

Moss R and Abdullayev F (2006) 'Saffron: Can it Cure Cancer? Scientists Are Convinced of Its Potency'. *Azerbaijan International*. Summer 14(2): 30–7. www.azer.com/aiweb/categories/magazine/ai142_folder/142_articles/142_saffron.html

Abdullaev FI (2002) 'Cancer Chemopreventive and Tumoricidal Properties of Saffron (Crocus sativus L.)'. *Experimental Biology and Medicine*. 227(1): 20. www.ebm.rsmjournals.com/cgi/reprint/227/1/20

Swiss Chard

Wood, R (1988) *The Whole Foods Encyclopedia*. New York, NY: Prentice-Hall Press.

Yanardag R, Bolkent S, Ozsoy-Sacan O et al. (2002) 'The effects of chard (Beta vulgaris L. var. cicla) extract on the kidney tissue, serum urea and creatinine levels of diabetic rats'. *Phytotherapy Research*. 16(8): 758–61.

Tomatoes

Béliveau, R and Gingras, D (2007) *Foods to Fight Cancer*. London: Dorling Kindersley.

Pratt S and Matthews K (2006) *SuperFoods Healthstyle, Proven Strategy for Lifelong Health*. London: Bantam.

Servan-Schreiber D (2008) *Anti-Cancer: A New Way of Life*. London: Michael Joseph.

Yellow Split Peas

Higdon J (2005) 'Whole Grains'. Micronutrient Information Center, Linus Pauling Institute, Oregon State University. www.lpi.oregonstate.edu/infocenter/foods/grains/

Mellitus MC, Garg A, Lutjohann D, Von Bergmann K, Grundy SM and Brinkley LJ (2000) 'Beneficial effects of high dietary fibre intake in patients with Type 2 Diabetes'. *The New England Journal of Medicine*. 342: 1392–98.

Index

Index

Index

Index